# INTERMITTENT FASTING
## FOR HUNGRY PEOPLE

MICHELLE STACEY

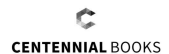

**CENTENNIAL** BOOKS

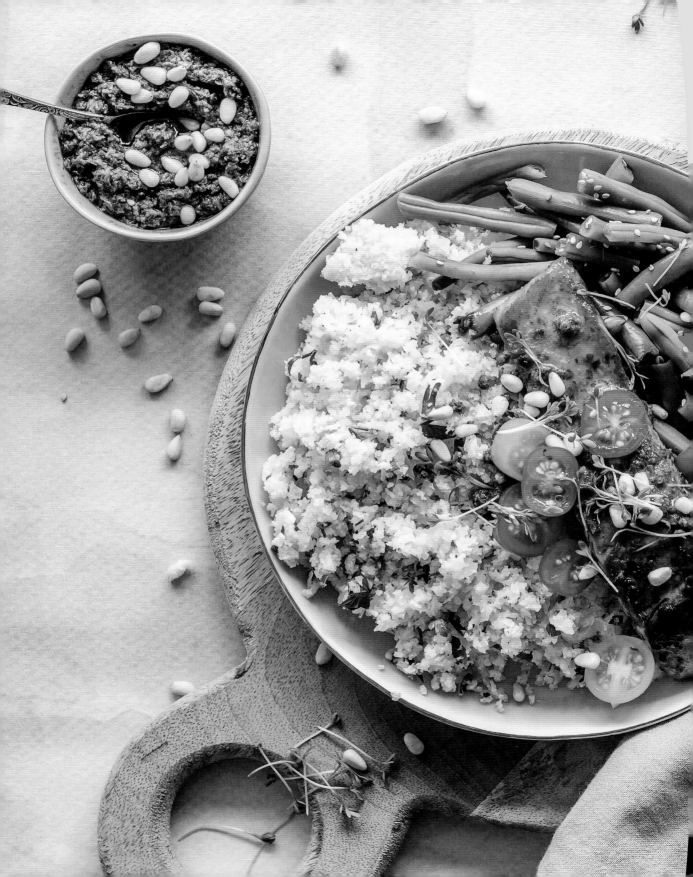

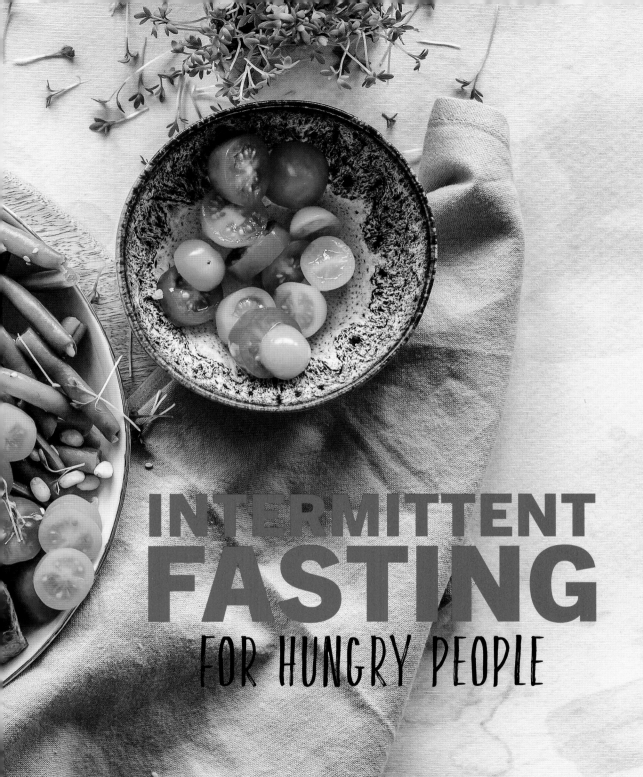

# INTERMITTENT FASTING

## FOR HUNGRY PEOPLE

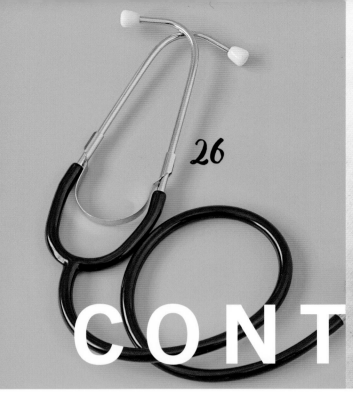

26

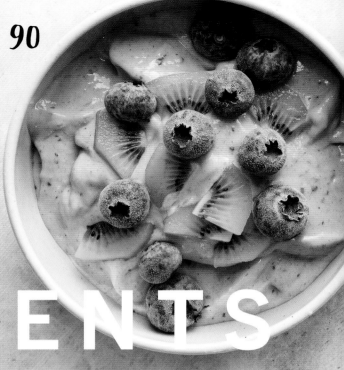

90

# CONTENTS

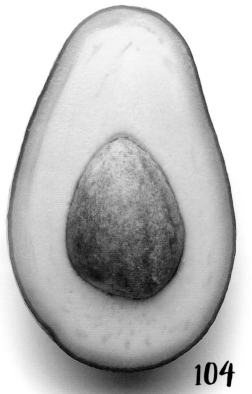

104

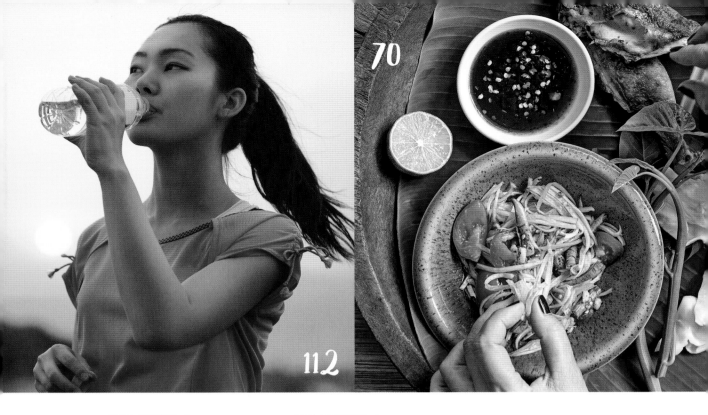

70

112

156

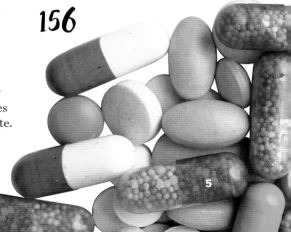

# LIFE IN THE
# FAST
# LANE

**Looking to lose weight, increase energy and improve your focus? Intermittent fasting may provide the answers— and it's far more enjoyable than you may think.**

**IF THERE'S A** holy grail of dieting, it might be this: a plan that lets you eat what you want, without tracking calories or outlawing favorite foods, and still helps you lose weight. For good measure, this diet also enhances your health, reducing your risk of certain chronic diseases, raising your metabolism and even helping to sharpen your mental clarity. To an increasing number of people, intermittent fasting may be the answer.

While "fasting" and "eating what you want" sound mutually exclusive, more and more research is showing that alternating between the two states works a surprising kind of magic. It's a deceptively simple concept, but goes against most current dieting wisdom: Instead of noshing on healthy snacks and never skipping a meal, you go for periods of time without eating anything at all. That can sound alarming to some, until you dig deeper into how intermittent fasting actually works.

For one thing, there's hunger. That's the most common fear about trying a fasting plan—and while at the beginning you will sometimes feel hungry, the human body has a powerful and complicated mechanism for moderating, and even nixing, hunger over time. Surprisingly, research shows you're unlikely to binge or overeat when you break your fast. Then there's your day-to-day lifestyle. How will you be able to have any kind of normal social life if you're living like a monk? Well, brace yourself: Breaking bread with friends can be easier to arrange on intermittent fasting than on a standard low-calorie diet.

As with all diets, there are optimal (and less-than-ideal) ways to go about intermittent fasting. This isn't a license to eat junk foods; the healthier you eat, the better your results will be. And, as with any plan, you'll need to find the form of fasting that works for you. This book will show you the way, from choosing between an alternate-day plan, one meal a day, or a daily "eating window" to mapping out the best meals and snacks for breaking the fast. It's also got important info about exercise, side effects, setbacks and plateaus. Read on for what you need to know to launch your fasting lifestyle—and start feeling stronger, healthier and more energetic than ever. —*Michelle Stacey*

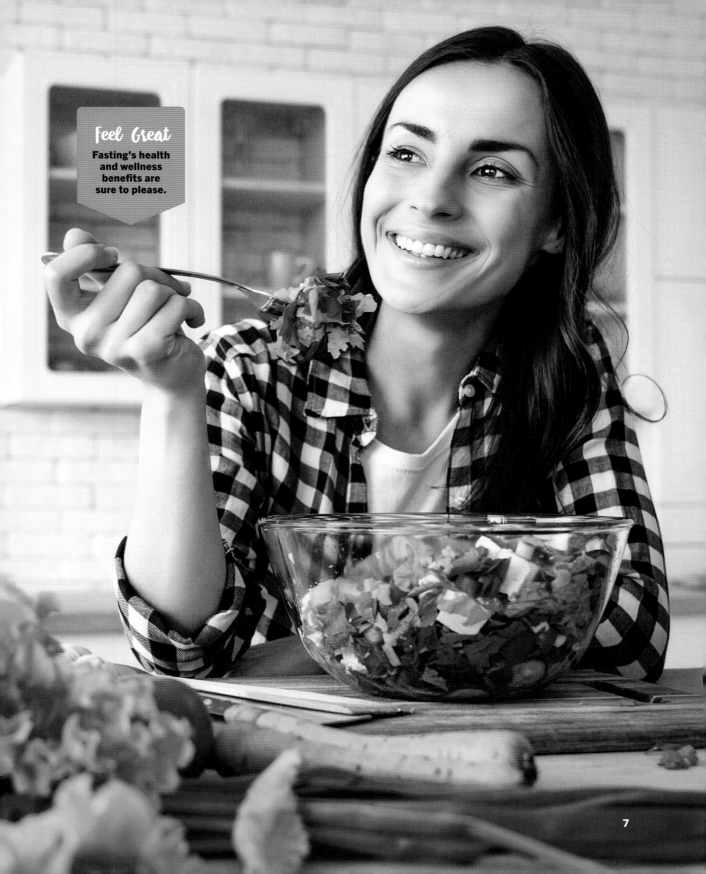

**Feel Great**
Fasting's health and wellness benefits are sure to please.

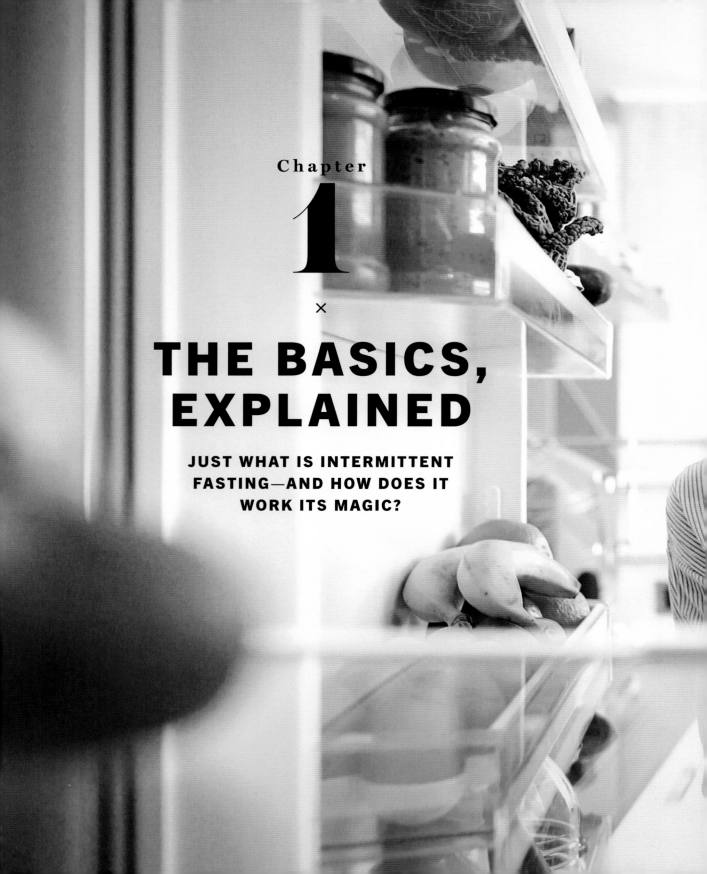

Chapter

# 1

×

# THE BASICS, EXPLAINED

## JUST WHAT IS INTERMITTENT FASTING—AND HOW DOES IT WORK ITS MAGIC?

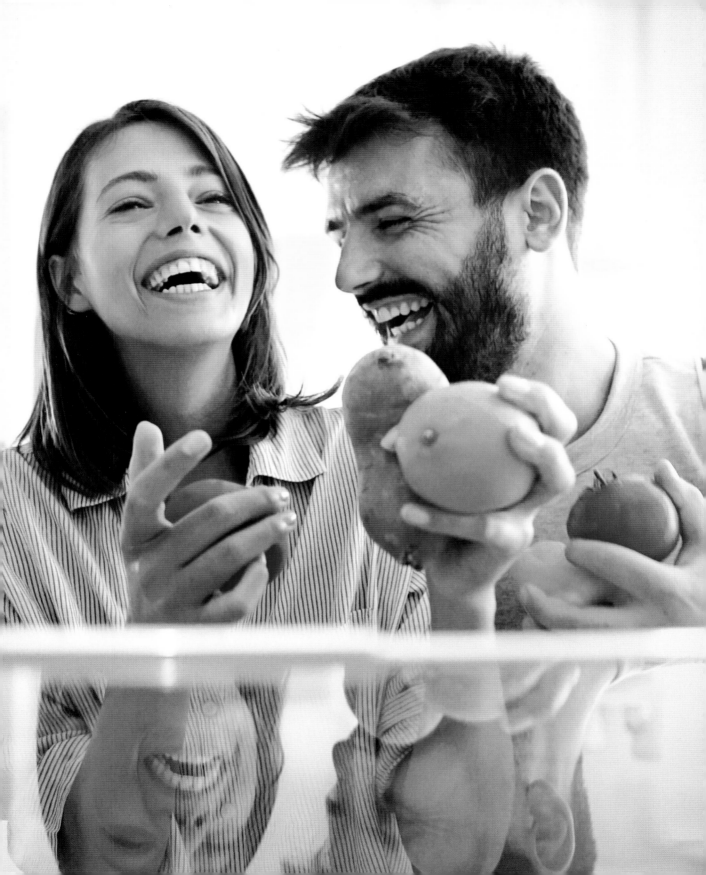

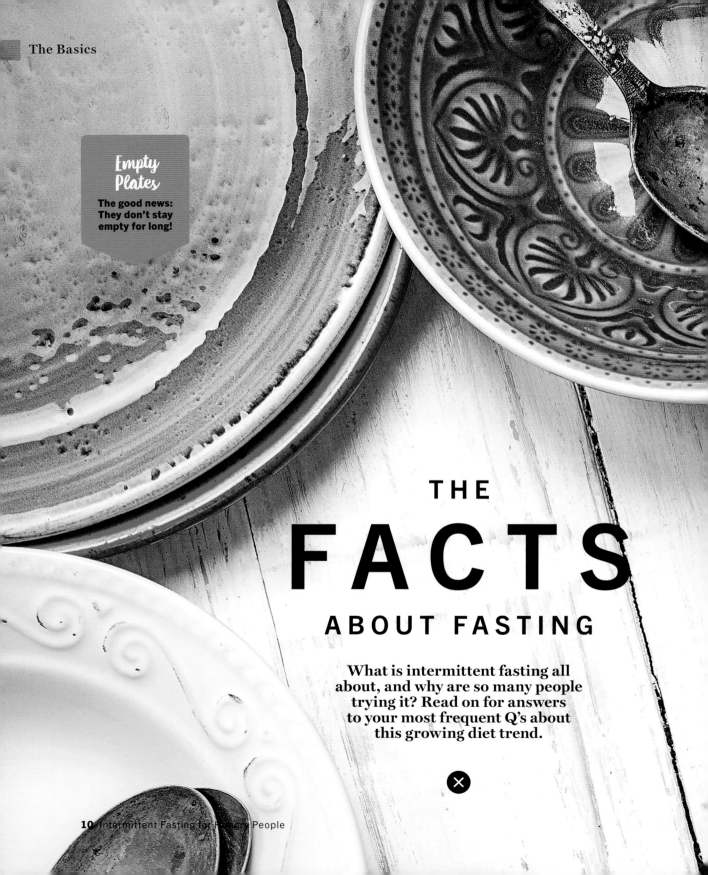

**Empty Plates**

The good news:
They don't stay
empty for long!

# THE
# FACTS
## ABOUT FASTING

What is intermittent fasting all
about, and why are so many people
trying it? Read on for answers
to your most frequent Q's about
this growing diet trend.

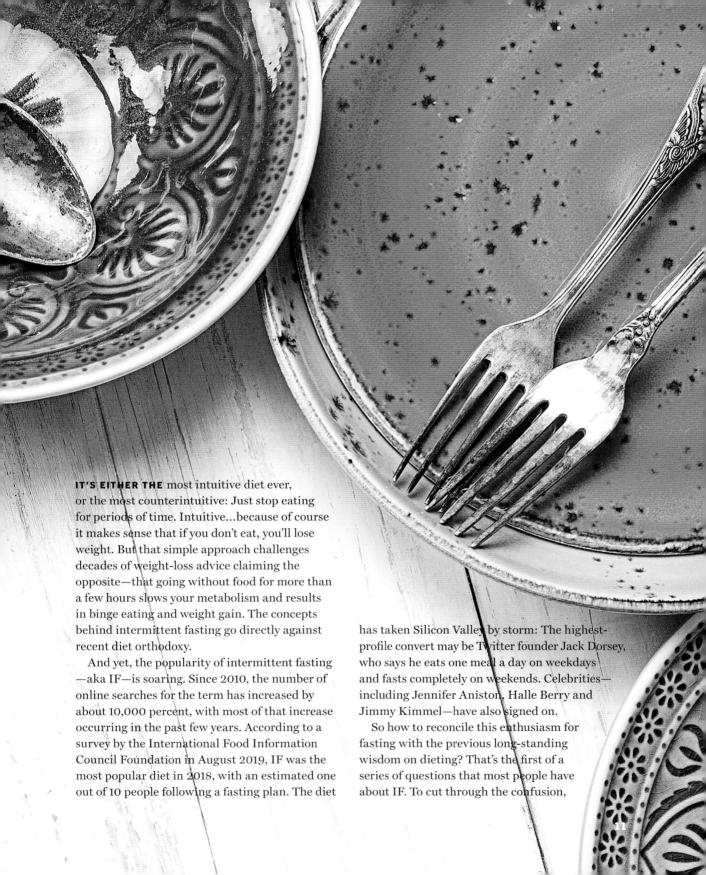

**IT'S EITHER THE** most intuitive diet ever, or the most counterintuitive: Just stop eating for periods of time. Intuitive...because of course it makes sense that if you don't eat, you'll lose weight. But that simple approach challenges decades of weight-loss advice claiming the opposite—that going without food for more than a few hours slows your metabolism and results in binge eating and weight gain. The concepts behind intermittent fasting go directly against recent diet orthodoxy.

And yet, the popularity of intermittent fasting —aka IF—is soaring. Since 2010, the number of online searches for the term has increased by about 10,000 percent, with most of that increase occurring in the past few years. According to a survey by the International Food Information Council Foundation in August 2019, IF was the most popular diet in 2018, with an estimated one out of 10 people following a fasting plan. The diet has taken Silicon Valley by storm: The highest-profile convert may be Twitter founder Jack Dorsey, who says he eats one meal a day on weekdays and fasts completely on weekends. Celebrities—including Jennifer Aniston, Halle Berry and Jimmy Kimmel—have also signed on.

So how to reconcile this enthusiasm for fasting with the previous long-standing wisdom on dieting? That's the first of a series of questions that most people have about IF. To cut through the confusion, let's take a look at some of the answers that have been emerging through both recent research and scads of anecdotal evidence.

## What Is IF?

At its most basic, intermittent fasting is choosing to restrict your eating—not by calorie-counting or by changing up the macronutrient content of your diet (i.e., going low-carb or low-fat) but simply by not eating for a predetermined amount of time. One common form of IF, for instance, is the 16:8 plan, in which you go without food for 16 hours at a stretch (seven or eight of which are usually spent sleeping) and eat all your calories within an eight-hour window. In real life, that could translate to skipping breakfast, eating at noon, and finishing dinner by 8 p.m. Other forms can involve abstaining from food (or reducing calories to 500 or so) for a day at a time, interspersed with days of normal eating. One example of that is the 5:2 plan—two days a week,

say Monday and Thursday, of fasting mixed in with five regular days. Yet another form is called one meal a day, or OMAD: fasting for most of the day, and clustering all of your calories into one big meal.

## Why Is It So Popular?

Fasting itself is not new at all. People have fasted for many reasons, from health to religion, for thousands of years (think of Yom Kippur, Lent or Ramadan). And the diet of prehistoric man included periods of food scarcity, suggesting that the human body is adapted to occasional fasts. But the recent iteration of fasting, with its focus on health and weight loss and its variety of approaches, was spurred by research into the effects of overall calorie restriction (called CR)—not slight calorie reduction, as in dieting, but cutting back on food intake, long term, by at least one-third. Studies in animals show that doing so makes them live longer, healthier lives. In humans, that level of food restriction (while not yet studied in the long term) produces similar health-promoting effects and lowers disease risk. The evidence is so strong that thousands of people (who call themselves CRONies, for Calorie Restriction with Optimum Nutrition) are living on severely restricted diets.

Not many of us, though, want to live on so little food. Enter IF, which research is showing can be similarly healthful—extending life and reducing disease risk—without slashing calories. "I was delighted to discover intermittent fasting," says Michael Mosley, MD, author of *The Fast Diet* and a long-term convert to the 5:2 plan. "It offered the benefits of CR but without the pain."

## How Hard Is It to Do?

That depends on who you ask. Mark Mattson, PhD, professor of neuroscience at Johns Hopkins University, has studied IF since the 1990s and has practiced it for years. "Once you get used to it, it's not a big deal," he says. "You adapt." Judging

### Cautionary Notes

For most people, fasting has been shown to be safe and beneficial. But there are a few situations where IF isn't wise.

**YOU SHOULDN'T FAST, IF YOU:**
* Are underweight
* Have a history of eating disorders like anorexia or bulimia
* Are pregnant or breastfeeding
* Are under the age of 18

**YOU CAN PROBABLY FAST, BUT MAY NEED MEDICAL SUPERVISION, IF YOU:**
* Have either Type 1 or Type 2 diabetes
* Take prescription medication
* Have gout or high uric acid levels
* Have a serious medical condition like liver, kidney or heart disease

13

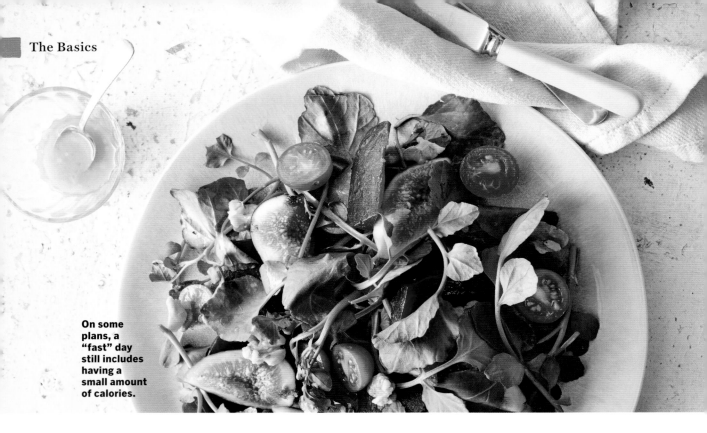

On some plans, a "fast" day still includes having a small amount of calories.

from the wave of social media (and celebrity) endorsements, many people agree. But it's not for everyone. A study in *JAMA Internal Medicine* compared IF followers to dieters restricting their daily calories by 25 percent and found they lost the same amount of weight and had similar reductions in cardiovascular risk factors like blood pressure, cholesterol and triglycerides.

However, the dropout rate in the IF group was 38 percent, versus 29 percent for the other dieters. It's worth noting that the IF protocol in the study was alternate-day fasting—eating only 25 percent of "energy needs" every other day—which many find harder than a 16:8 plan, where you eat every day within an eight-hour window.

## But Is It Safe?

Studies have found that, beyond being safe, IF has many benefits. A landmark study in 2008

✕

# OLD-THINK: EAT MANY SMALL MEALS PER DAY. NEW-THINK: THAT'S A RECIPE FOR OBESITY.

found that fasting for two days protected healthy cells against the toxicity of chemotherapy, while the cancer cells stayed sensitive. IF has also been shown to improve many health markers, including insulin sensitivity, blood pressure, cholesterol and overall disease risk. That said, check in with your doctor before starting IF, says Cary Kreutzer, RD, director of the Master of Science in Nutrition, Healthspan and Longevity program at the University of Southern California.

# Four Fasting Myths Debunked

Despite the growing popularity and increased acceptance of intermittent fasting for both weight loss and overall health, a variety of myths and fears about voluntarily pushing away the plate have persisted. Here are some of the most common misconceptions—and what you need to know.

## myth 1

### FASTING CAUSES LOW BLOOD SUGAR

Glucose derived from the breaking down of carbohydrate foods is your body's favorite fuel—but *not* its only fuel. "People think their bodies will deplete themselves of all the food energy that's currently available," says Megan Ramos, co-founder of the Intensive Dietary Management Program, an online nutrition consulting firm. "What they don't understand is that we have mechanisms that store food energy, and that can retrieve it when we need it." When you fast, not only can your body turn to stored fat for fuel, but counterregulatory hormones also kick in to work against the action of insulin and raise blood glucose as needed. In addition, the liver is able to break down stored fat into ketones, and can even manufacture new glucose in a process called gluconeogenesis. Bottom line: Your body has amazing powers to keep you on an even keel and prevent signs of hypoglycemia like shakiness and lightheadedness.

## myth 2

### FASTING WILL BURN YOUR MUSCLE MASS

If anything, fasting preserves muscle mass because of its effect on hormones like human growth hormone, says Ramos; what you burn instead is stored body fat. "Your body fat is your fuel reserve, while muscle mass is functional and serves a purpose, so why would you burn that? Imagine you're in a cabin during winter—are you going to chop up your sofa, which is functional, to build a fire, or are you going to burn the firewood that's stacked up on the porch to serve as fuel? That's your body fat."

## myth 3

### FASTING SLOWS YOUR METABOLISM

The opposite is true: A recent study in the journal *Scientific Reports* found that fasting may boost metabolic activity, especially in metabolites that are responsible for the maintenance of muscle, and other research has shown metabolic benefits from time-restricted (16:8) fasting. Traditional diets do slow metabolism (as was demonstrated in a study of weight regain among *The Biggest Loser* contestants), because your body learns how to subsist on fewer calories over time by slowing the rate at which you burn calories. But when you remove *all* food for periods of time, a number of mechanisms kick in (including changes in hormones and mitochondria, the energy "factories" in your cells) that help your body plunder fuel from your fat stores.

## myth 4

### FASTING MAKES YOU BINGE LATER

That seems so logical —wouldn't you stuff your face after being deprived for 16 hours to a day or more? But it's simply not true. Studies show that calorie intake does go up a bit after a fast, but quickly settles back down, resulting in an overall calorie deficit over time. That may be due at least in part to changes in hunger hormones like ghrelin and leptin; over time, ghrelin (an appetite-boosting hormone) declines when fasting. "The first time I did a three-day fast, I had planned a big romantic dinner to end the fast," says Ramos. "Then I could hardly eat it. I just didn't have the hunger."

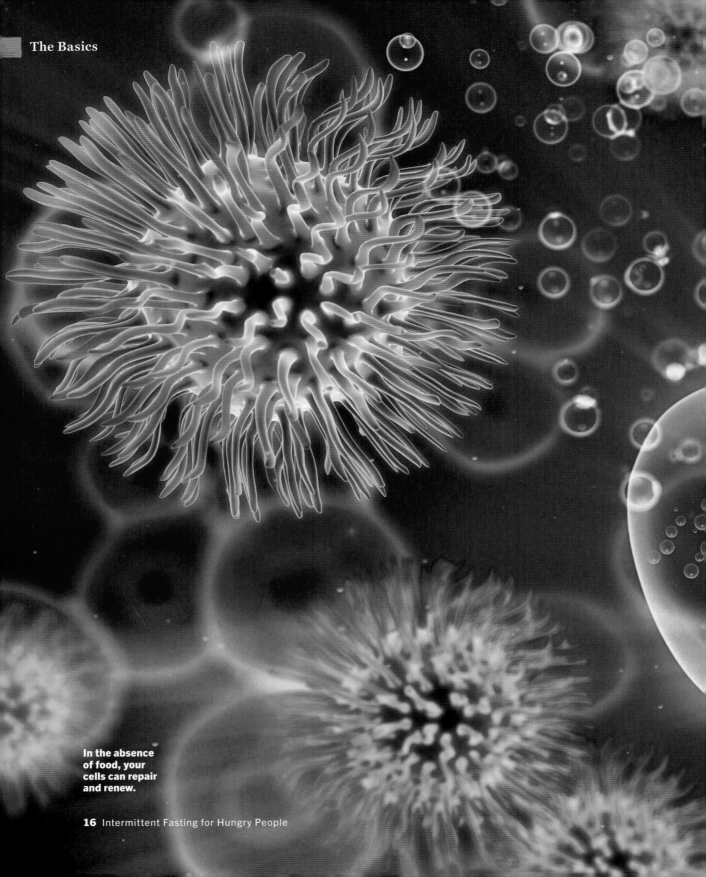

In the absence
of food, your
cells can repair
and renew.

# THE
# SCIENCE
## BEHIND IT

Growing evidence shows that fasting
affects your body right down to the cellular level.
Read the latest about its inner workings.

✕

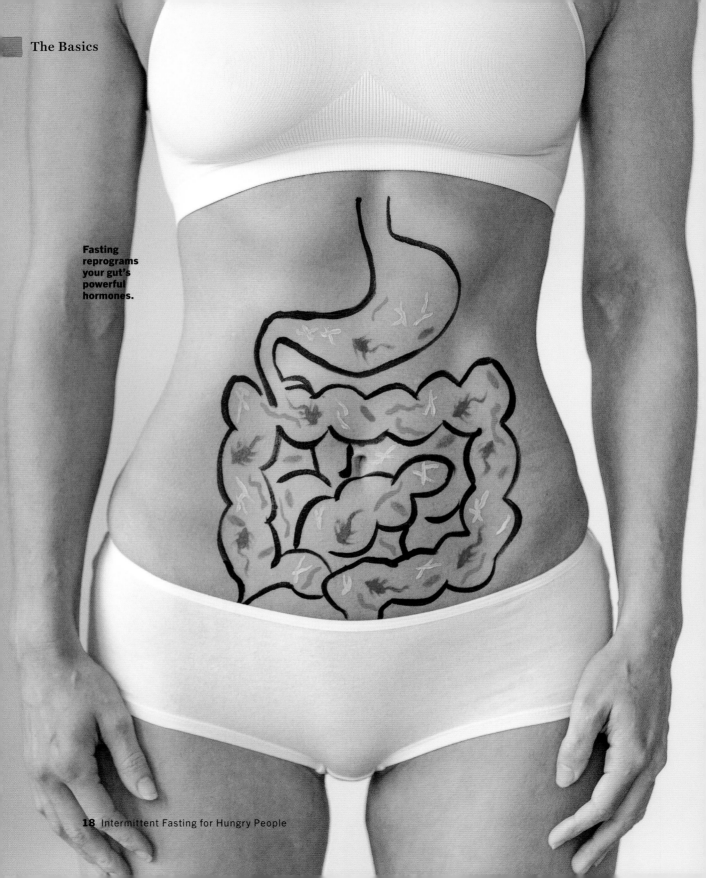

**Fasting reprograms your gut's powerful hormones.**

**IN ONE WAY,** intermittent fasting is simple to define: You stop eating for a preplanned period of time. But reams of research are demonstrating that doing so spurs a series of complex reactions in your body, from the functioning of certain organs to the behavior of cells, hormones and blood proteins. In order to understand how and why IF may not only help you lose weight, but also make you stronger and healthier, you need to take a deep dive into your body's physiology. What you'll find: some profound effects of the decision to, for example, not eat your breakfast until noon. Here's what happens.

## Where It Started

First, a little evolutionary history: How did humans eat long ago, when our bodies were laying down the basic biology that exists to this day? Anthropologists posit that before the modern era, intermittent fasting happened not infrequently, and out of necessity. Food supplies were often unreliable, especially as you look back into prehistory when our forebears were hunters and gatherers, before agriculture began about 12,000

years ago. Famine was often hovering, whether for a few days or an entire season.

That fact may help explain how the human body responds to a fast today, says Jason Fung, MD, author of *The Complete Guide to Fasting*. "It makes a lot of sense from an evolutionary standpoint," he says. "Animals that are cognitively sharp and physically agile during times of food scarcity have a clear advantage when it comes to survival." If, on the other hand, missing a meal or two made you weak, confused or fatigued, you would have even more trouble finding food— not a good thing for the survival of the species.

As agriculture helped assure a more steady food supply (though not nearly as steady as the always-available food culture that exists today, at least in developed countries), ancient civilizations like the Greeks began to incorporate voluntary fasting into their lives. "The Greeks recognized there was something deeply, intrinsically beneficial to periodic fasting," says Fung. He considers fasting "the most time-honored and widespread healing tradition in the world."

One other thing to know about our bodies' familiarity with fasting, Fung adds, is that until about the 1980s, people naturally incorporated periods of fasting into their daily lives without even realizing it. A typical day's eating in the

A review found an average loss of 7 to 11 pounds over 10 weeks for those on a fasting diet.

✕

## INSULIN IS ESSENTIAL TO LIFE, BUT IN OUR CONSTANT-NOSHING WORLD TODAY, IT HAS BECOME OVERUSED.

✕

## LONG BEFORE MICROSCOPES AND MRIs, THE ANCIENTS SAW THAT FASTING BOOSTED BRAIN POWER.

1970s, he says, might include breakfast at 8 a.m., lunch at noon, and dinner at 6 p.m.—and snacking was not encouraged. "That means we would be eating for 10 hours of the day, nicely balanced by 14 hours of fasting." Studies have supported this; one in the *American Journal of Clinical Nutrition* (*AJCN*) found that over the past 30 years the time between "eating occasions" declined for both adults and children, meaning that across the board, Americans "are consuming food more frequently throughout the day." And over that same period, perhaps not coincidentally, the number of Americans who are overweight or obese has increased dramatically.

### The Insulin Connection

Studies have shown all kinds of benefits of IF, from improvements in markers in heart health and blood sugar to weight loss and anti-aging effects. But what makes these happen? The first answer ties directly to the increase in eating occasions shown in the *AJCN* study. Your body basically exists in two states: fed and fasted, explains Ted Naiman, MD, co-author of *The P:E Diet*. When you eat (and for hours afterward), you're in the fed state, in which your body releases insulin from the pancreas. Insulin functions as a key to open your cells, so the calories you're taking in can enter and your body can be fueled. But insulin doesn't just enable this transfer; it also functions as essentially a fat-storage hormone, putting any excess calories quickly into the fat cells. In the presence of insulin, the burning of

fat is halted, says Naiman, while the body uses glucose (from your last meal) instead.

The fed state, followed by what's called the fasted (postabsorptive) state, lasts around 12 hours. At that point, you run out of glucose from the meal you ate, and your insulin has fallen precipitously. With fat-storing insulin out of the way, your fat cells unlock and allow your body to start burning fat for fuel until you eat again. A simple way to think about it, says Naiman, is that "you can only burn stored body fat while in the fasted state, and you can only store more body fat while in the fed state." So imagine you have a post-dinner snack—say, cookies or popcorn—at 9 or 10 o'clock, and then eat a breakfast muffin or toast at 7 or 8 in the morning. Your body has been

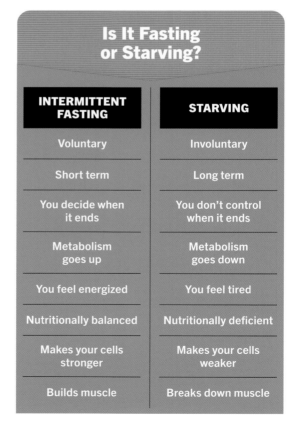

| Is It Fasting or Starving? | |
| --- | --- |
| **INTERMITTENT FASTING** | **STARVING** |
| Voluntary | Involuntary |
| Short term | Long term |
| You decide when it ends | You don't control when it ends |
| Metabolism goes up | Metabolism goes down |
| You feel energized | You feel tired |
| Nutritionally balanced | Nutritionally deficient |
| Makes your cells stronger | Makes your cells weaker |
| Builds muscle | Breaks down muscle |

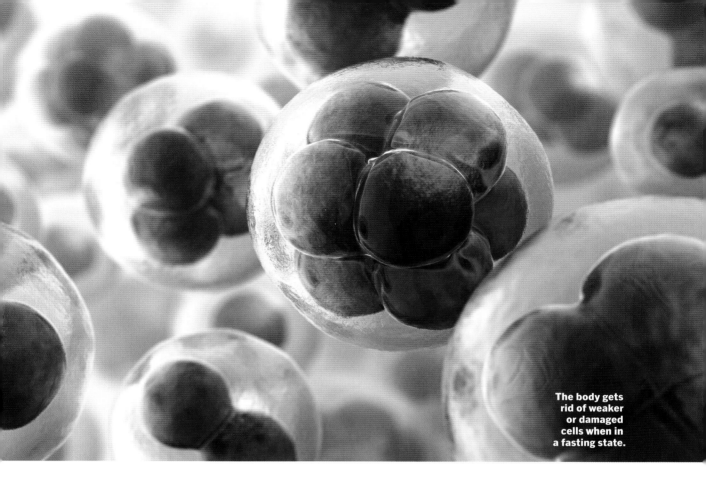

The body gets rid of weaker or damaged cells when in a fasting state.

happily feasting on glucose that whole time, with any excess safely tucked away in your fat cells. And before it has a chance to unlock those fat cells, it gets more glucose. The fat storage continues, and the number on your scale continues to rise.

Over time, if the body is in the fed state often (those many eating occasions), the mitochondria—or tiny energy factories inside the cells—develop a preference for the easily accessed glucose from food. They prefer it over fat, which is harder to break down, so when you run out of fuel because insulin has stored so much of it away, instead of burning stored fat you get hungry for more food. Another result of frequent feeding is that your insulin stays high, eventually leading to insulin resistance and, in increasing numbers of people, Type 2 diabetes.

Adding periods of abstaining from food, on the other hand, lets you enter the fasting state and start burning fat.

## Cell Repair

Insulin resistance has been linked to a number of health issues, including heart disease, stroke, high blood pressure, abdominal obesity and many others—so putting your body into a low-insulin state on a regular basis helps lower your risk of these conditions. But fasting has also been shown to help your body repair itself, much as you might take your aging car in for some new parts, and this is also connected to insulin levels. To stay healthy, your body must constantly "cleanse" your cells through a process called autophagy (in Greek, autophagy literally means "self-eating"). This involves getting rid of diseased or broken-down cellular components, explains Fung.

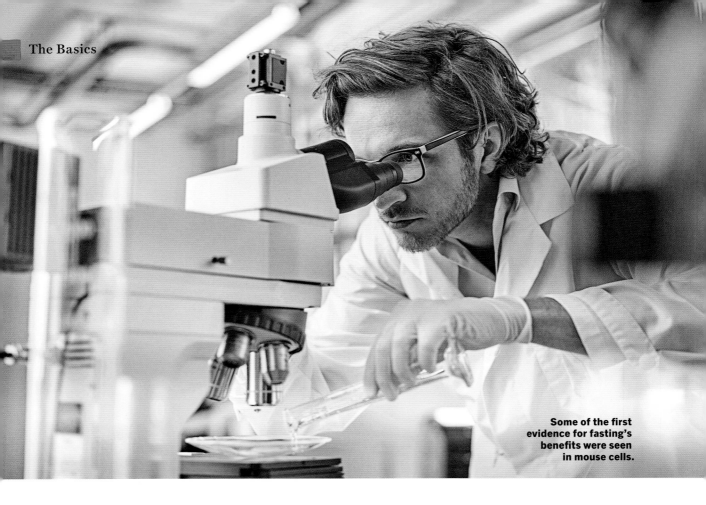

**Some of the first evidence for fasting's benefits were seen in mouse cells.**

Only after these nonworking parts have been cleared out can your body renew itself, he adds.

But here's the catch: Increased levels of glucose, insulin and proteins from food all turn off autophagy. So, says Fung, "by eating constantly, from the time we wake up to the time we sleep, we prevent the activation of autophagy's cleansing pathways. Simply put, fasting cleanses the body of unhealthy or unnecessary cellular debris." This helps explain why many studies show a link between IF and a lower risk of dementia (which is caused in part by cellular "debris" in the brain), as well as a slowing of aging in general. It also explains why fasting has often been characterized as cleansing or purifying, even by ancient populations.

In a related way, fasting also stimulates the release of growth hormone, which helps build new replacement cells for the ones that have been "eaten" in autophagy. Growth hormone is only released in the absence of insulin, says Naiman. In fact, overeating can suppress growth hormone levels by as much as 80 percent. On the other hand, "growth hormone rises by as much as 2,000 percent after 24 hours of fasting," says Naiman (although it starts rising even before that).

Human growth hormone, or HGH, has been marketed as an anti-aging supplement, but taking it as a supplement has side effects. Regular periods of fasting appear to be a way to get the cellular and anti-aging benefits naturally, says Fung. While low levels of growth hormone in adults lead to more body fat and less muscle mass, higher levels do the opposite—helping to build muscle and burn fat. "Many of the effects of aging may result from low growth hormone levels," Fung says. It makes evolutionary sense that fasting builds muscle, Naiman adds: "In our ancestors, if going without food made you weaker and slower you would never find more food. Humans would have been extinct."

## Inside the Brain

One common assumption about fasting is that it must somehow make you mentally sluggish—after all, our brains need constant food, right? But not only do many people anecdotally say they actually feel sharper and more focused while fasting (one reason IF is a hit among Silicon Valley types), studies in both animals and humans support this. Researchers say there may be multiple mechanisms for this "brain boost." One involves a protein called brain-derived neurotrophic factor (BDNF), which is essential to brain function and the development of neurons—and which gets boosted by fasting. Problems with BDNF signaling are involved in several neurodegenerative disorders, including Alzheimer's disease. BDNF prompts the growth of new neurons in the hippocampus, the brain region involved in learning and memory, a process called neuroplasticity.

A major review of the evidence on IF, published in *Nature Reviews Neuroscience* in 2018, found that IF "impacts multiple signaling pathways that promote neuroplasticity and resistance of the brain to injury and disease." Again, this makes evolutionary sense: Early humans whose brains worked well during famines were more likely to find food and survive to reproduce.

Fasting's brain benefits may also be due to ketones, an alternative fuel source made by the liver when glucose runs low. The brain can only be fueled by glucose or ketones, not directly by fat. And many scientists feel that ketones are a superior fuel that burns more "cleanly."

One other reason IF ups brain function involves reducing inflammation, which is key to brain

×

# RATHER THAN FEELING FUZZY, PEOPLE ON A FAST REPORT AN INCREASE IN THEIR ABILITY TO FOCUS.

health. Inflammation has been linked to various psychiatric disorders, as well as neurodegenerative diseases like Alzheimer's. Some studies show a reduction of inflammation among fasters. Lower inflammation goes hand in hand with autophagy, which clears your brain circuits of damaged cells so neurons can communicate.

## Your Inner Motor

Many people fear that going without food for more than a few hours will make their metabolism—the rate at which your body burns calories—begin to slow down. It's been shown that dieting can indeed slow your metabolism;

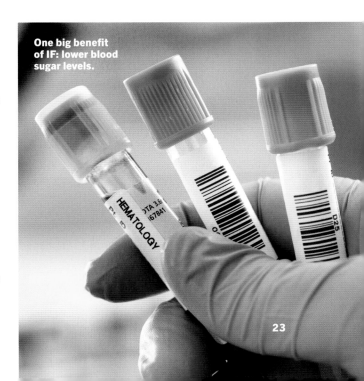

One big benefit of IF: lower blood sugar levels.

that's one reason so many contestants on the show *The Biggest Loser* later regained most of the weight they lost. But there's a big difference between simply lowering overall calories while eating regularly throughout the day, and gathering all your calories into a small window of "eating occasions," and it involves that powerful fat-storing hormone, insulin.

Every time you eat, insulin is released and locks up your fat stores. If you're noshing frequently, your insulin level never drops enough for you to start burning fat. The result: your metabolism slows so that you can make better use of the calories you *do* bring in. But when you fast—whether for an occasional day, or for 14 to 16 hours of each day—your insulin goes down and your body can burn

## Your Brain on Fasting

Far from feeling lightheaded or fuzzy, you're more likely to get a burst of mental clarity during a fast. Here's why.

If there's a reason Silicon Valley whizzes have embraced IF, it may be in part because of fasting's profound impact on brain function. Studies have shown several different cellular mechanisms that may account for IF's apparent brain benefits. One is autophagy, which may help clear cellular debris that could disrupt communication between synapses. A major review of the evidence at the U.S. National Institute on Aging, published in *Nature Reviews Neuroscience*, found

that IF "impacts multiple signaling pathways that promote neuroplasticity and resistance of the brain to injury and disease."

Ketone bodies that are produced through fasting also appear to have specific benefits to the brain, according to Shelly Fan, PhD. The brain can use only glucose or ketones as fuel (fat can't cross the blood-brain barrier), and "some types of ketones may be more efficient as fuel than glucose," says Fan. "Fasting also tells the cells to synthesize more

mitochondria—our cellular energy factories." The more mitochondria you have, the more efficient the energy supply to the brain. That may help explain why many fasters say they feel particularly sharp and focused while abstaining from food.

One more factor in the IF-brain health connection: a protein called brain-derived neurotrophic factor, or BDNF, which is essential to brain function and prompts the growth of new neurons in the hippocampus, the center of learning and memory. BDNF dysfunction has been linked to several neurodegenerative disorders, including Alzheimer's. A study in the *Annual Review of Nutrition*, among others, found that IF increased the production of BDNF, which in turn boosted the resistance of neurons in the brain to dysfunction. All of these brain benefits show the wisdom of Mother Nature: When our ancestors were low on fuel, their brain power kicked in to help them survive a famine and find new sources of food.

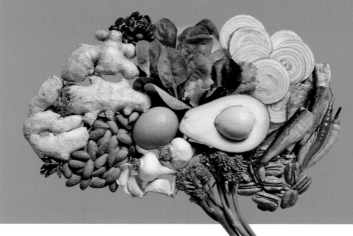

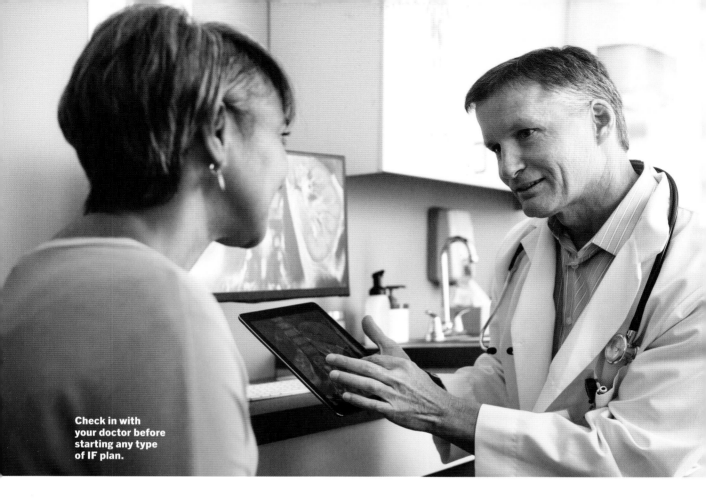

Check in with your doctor before starting any type of IF plan.

stored fat. There's no reason to slow metabolism to conserve energy, so it keeps humming along.

## A Little Stress

Most of these mechanisms illustrate one truth about the human body: A little bit of stress is a good thing. Put another way, what does not kill you makes you stronger. It's a principle called hormesis, and it's the reason cardio exercise strengthens your heart and resistance training strengthens your muscles. When you exercise, you're doing a little bit of damage to your body, stressing it out by making it work harder for a period of time and causing microscopic rips and tears. When you stop, your body goes into recovery mode, and that's when actual progress is made—repair genes get switched on, and your muscles get patched up in a way that increases their size and strength.

Hormesis is the process that makes a plant create more branches and flowers after it is cut back; the plant suffers stress, prompting it to work harder to stay strong. You can even apply it to emotions: Going through something difficult strengthens you for the next time. "Hormesis is now a well-accepted biological explanation of how things operate at the cellular level," says Michael Mosley, MD, author of *The Fast Diet*. And, he adds, many researchers feel that hormesis is at the heart of why intermittent fasting has so many benefits throughout the body. IF puts your cells under minor stress, and they get stronger: "The challenge itself is part of the benefit," says Mosley. And the best news, as many intermittent fasters are finding, is that the "challenge" of going without food for a limited time is not very hard at all.

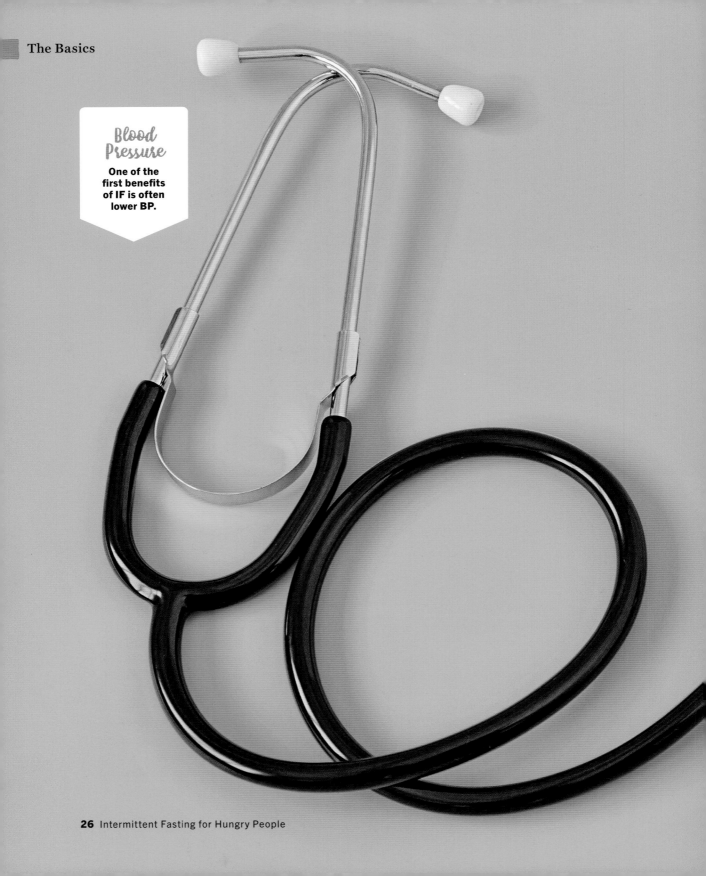

*Blood Pressure*

**One of the first benefits of IF is often lower BP.**

# THE
# HEALTH
## PAYOFF

**The complicated workings of intermittent fasting deep inside your cells add up to concrete benefits in how your body functions. And weight loss is just the beginning.**

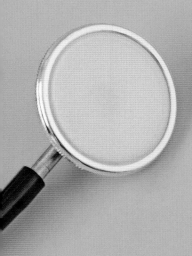

**WHEN INTERMITTENT FASTING** works its magic by altering your body's use of insulin, there's a ripple effect: lower heart disease risk, improved blood sugar control, more definitive weight loss. And reducing inflammation and increasing growth hormone levels increases your odds of living longer and avoiding dementia. Research has revealed a trove of physical and mental benefits as a result of what IF does in your body on a molecular level. Here are five ways it can help.

## Weight Loss

The hope of dropping pounds is what prompts many people to try IF, often before they realize that fasting has other benefits. In a 2014 review published in *Translational Research*, IF was found to reduce body weight by 3 to 8 percent over a period of three to 24 weeks. Another meta-analysis published in the *Journal of the Academy of Nutrition and Dietetics* found that "almost any intermittent-fasting regimen can result in weight loss." And a third research review, published in the journal *Cureus*, concluded IF was "efficient in reducing weight" and that people on it showed "significant decrease in fat mass."

Other research has looked at specific types of IF, with similar results. A study in *Diabetologia* found that eating the same number of calories in two meals a day—breakfast and lunch—rather than in six smaller ones led to lower body weight and greater fat loss. And it doesn't have to be those two meals; a study in *BMJ* showed that people who skipped breakfast weighed less and took in fewer calories than those who ate breakfast daily. Both patterns follow the 16:8 "time window" approach of eating all calories within eight hours per day, and both were effective. Alternate-day fasting, akin to the 5:2 pattern of fasting two days a week, was also shown to boost weight loss and lower fat in a study in *Obesity Reviews*.

Monique Tello, MD, MPH, a physician at Massachusetts General Hospital, relates how she was once a skeptic about IF, only to be convinced by the evidence. "I had written off IF as no better or worse than simply eating less," she says. After reading recent studies, though, she now feels "there is good scientific evidence suggesting that circadian rhythm fasting [the 16:8 plan] can be an effective approach to weight loss."

But science has shown that many diets provoke weight loss—at least for a time. What might make IF superior? One answer is that it may cause weight loss without restricting calories, says Satchidananda Panda, PhD, a professor at the Salk Institute for Biological Studies in La Jolla, California. In one study, Panda and his team split mice into two groups. One ate unrestricted sugary, fatty foods during a 24-hour period; the other ate the same foods but only during an eight-hour window (the 16:8 plan). All the mice ate the same number of calories, but the constant eaters became fat and sick, and the 16:8 mice did not. Similar evidence has researchers thinking that weight control is not just calories in/calories out, and that timing influences how our bodies deal with calories.

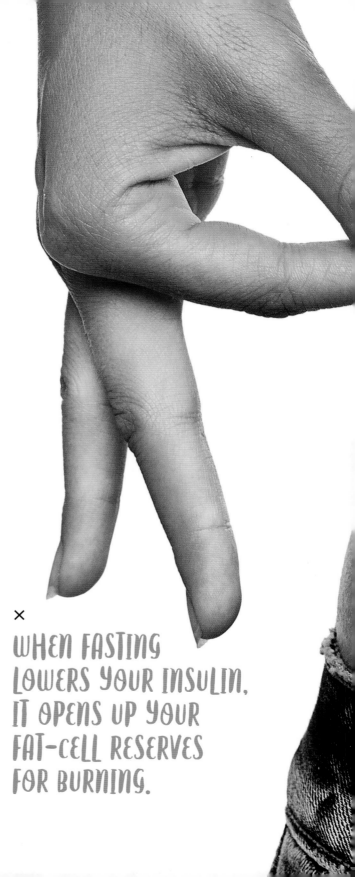

✕

WHEN FASTING LOWERS YOUR INSULIN, IT OPENS UP YOUR FAT-CELL RESERVES FOR BURNING.

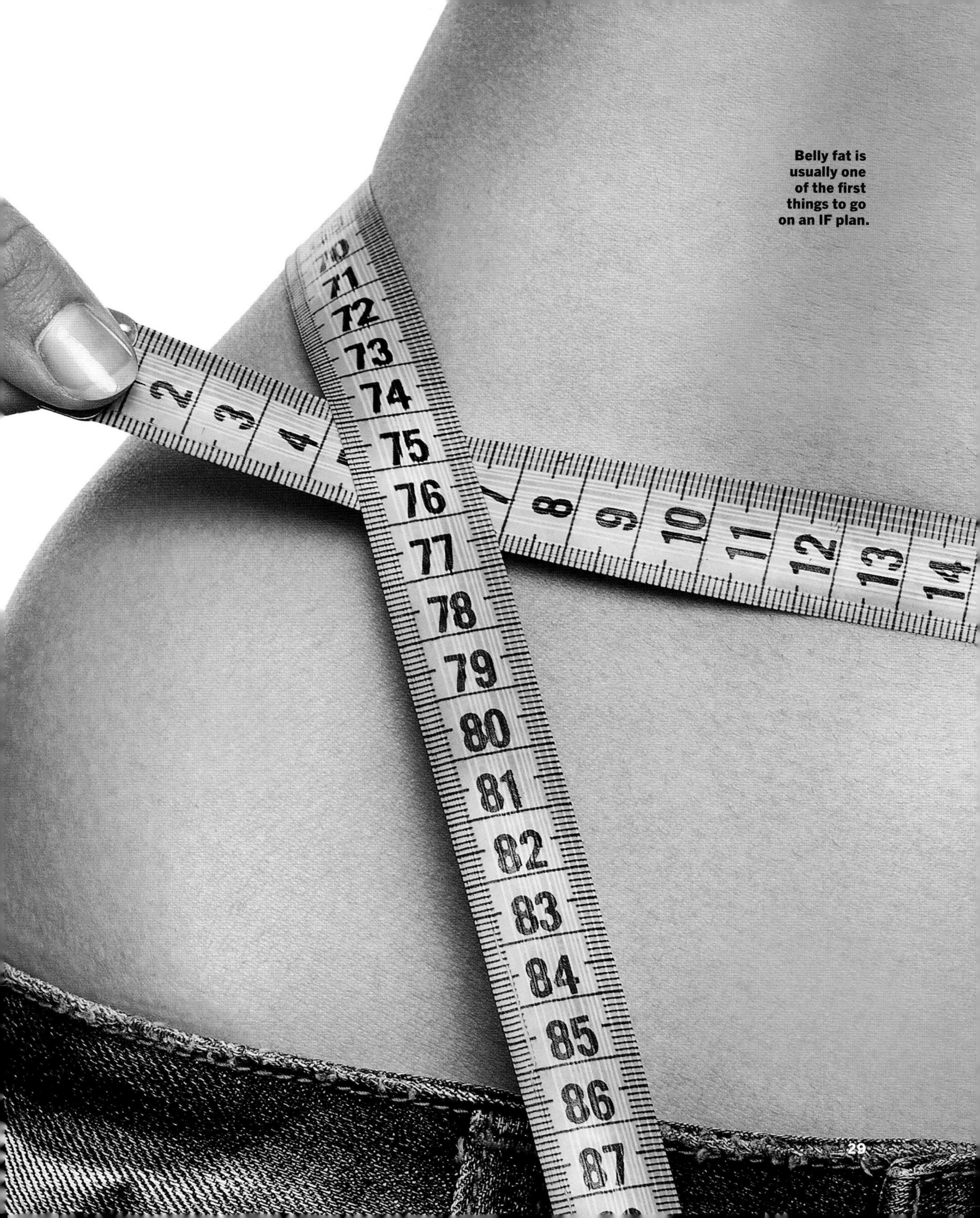

Belly fat is
usually one
of the first
things to go
on an IF plan.

"What we can say for sure is that overweight humans who switch their eating pattern to IF and stick with it will have a lower body weight with lower fat stores and better glucose regulation," says Mark Mattson, PhD, who has studied IF for decades.

## Stable Blood Sugar

That "glucose regulation" Mattson mentions is one key to how IF achieves its weight-loss wonders. Studies have shown that any form of IF has a powerful effect on how your body releases and uses insulin, and how much glucose you have in your blood. When you eat often, your pancreas keeps secreting insulin, which lets the glucose from food into your cells (and is very efficient at storing extra calories and locking them away in your fat cells). If you have a "grazing" dietary habit—even if it's healthy food—eventually your cells become less responsive to insulin because it's ever-present. So you produce even more insulin, entering a cycle of blood sugar and insulin peaks

# YOUR BODY GETS BUSY WHEN FASTING, CLEANING OUT DAMAGED CELLS.

that can result in obesity, insulin resistance, diabetes, and even heart disease and stroke.

But if you take periodic breaks from food—whether it's 16 hours out of every day, or a full fasting day or two per week—your insulin falls, blood sugar stabilizes and your fat stores unlock. "Regularly lowering insulin levels leads to improved insulin sensitivity," says Jason Fung, MD. One study that convinced Tello of IF's efficacy involved obese men with prediabetes: One group ate all their meals within eight hours, and the other ate their calories over 12 hours. Both groups maintained the same weight, but after five weeks, the eight-hour men had lower insulin levels and

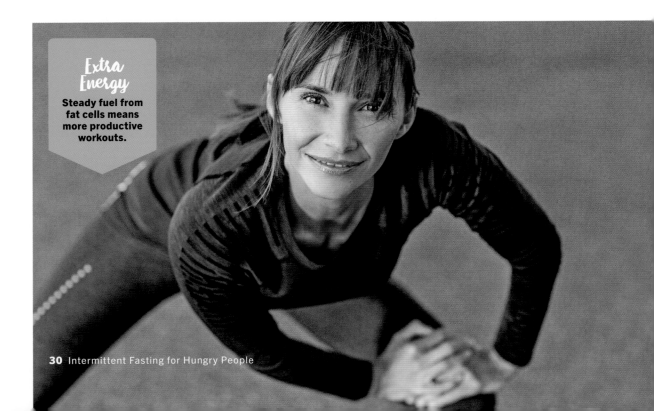

### Extra Energy
**Steady fuel from fat cells means more productive workouts.**

much-improved insulin sensitivity. "The best part was that the eight-hour group also had decreased appetite," says Tello. "They weren't starving." Other studies have shown similar benefits.

## A Stronger Heart

Many studies that show weight loss and better insulin control with IF also show changes in markers that affect heart disease and stroke risk: lower blood pressure and decreases in LDL cholesterol (the bad kind) and triglycerides. That's not surprising, considering that both obesity and insulin resistance are implicated in cardiovascular disease—they're all connected at a cellular level.

Panda has conducted studies with fruit flies (because their hearts are similar to ours) on a time-restricted eating plan, and found that their hearts appeared 20 to 30 percent younger than their age. "It works by keeping the heart's mitochondria healthy, which reduces oxidative stress," Panda said, adding that time-restricted eating gives the body time to repair itself. "Most of our studies show that the effect is on multiple organs and on the central nervous system. It's a positive-feedback loop."

## A Clearer Head

Fasting has a reputation for being a "brain booster," and research is beginning to show just how that may account for a clearer head. Mattson explains that fasting puts cells in a "stress-resistance mode" in which they clean house, removing damaged molecules and proteins through a process called autophagy. "Then, during the resting or refeeding period, once the cell has cleared out the garbage, protein synthesis goes up and new proteins are created. We have evidence that this doesn't just benefit muscle cells—in the brain, new synapses may be formed between nerve cells."

Animal studies bear this out: Aging rats put on IF regimens markedly improved their motor coordination, cognition, learning and memory. Human studies on caloric restriction find similar neurologic benefits, says Fung, and "this is one area where fasting and caloric reduction provide similar benefits." When insulin goes lower, memory improves. One more connection: A higher body mass index is linked to a decline in mental abilities and less blood flow to the area of the brain involved in attention, focus, reasoning and abstract thought.

## A Longer Life

Almost all of these positive effects of fasting come together in one big takeaway, say researchers: IF may not only extend your life, but make those extra years healthier. Much of that effect, says Mattson, is due to autophagy, the process that "cleans out" old, damaged cells so that new, healthy cells can replace them. And with IF's boost to your growth hormone levels, you're also able to make new cells, aiding your entire body. In addition, fasting reduces inflammation, a driver of aging. Research shows that animals on long-term dietary restriction can survive 60 percent longer, with few chronic diseases and a slowed rate of aging. Humans may also gain years from IF, say experts, simply by periodically restricting calories.

---

## A Faster Metabolism
### Unlike other plans, IF may boost your burn rate.

**NOT YOUR USUAL DIET!**
With most low-calorie diets, metabolism plummets. But with IF "your body is still being fueled," says Jason Fung, MD. "It's just getting energy from burning stored body fat rather than food." Studies show that after fasting, energy expenditure can increase by up to 12 percent, making fasting a form of "metabolic exercise," according to Ted Naiman, MD. IF also increases adrenaline levels, which stimulates metabolism.

# YOUR BODY ON
# FASTING

**Whatever form you choose, intermittent fasting brings a full-figure transformation. Here's the anatomy of IF, from head to toe.**

**PICTURE THIS: YOUR** organs, bloodstream, hormones and your mitochondria—the energy factories within each cell—respond to every period of fasting you go through. Even a standard overnight fast, from dinner to breakfast (when you "break" your daily "fast"), produces changes and adjustments in how your body functions. The surprise to many is that these changes are positive ones. By timing your fasts in a way that still provides you with optimal nutrition, you skip any detriments that come with true starvation mode, and instead reap the benefits of our innate human physiology—one that has adapted through millennia to thrive through periods of food scarcity. This blueprint shows how it works.

### Brain

Studies show IF can prompt neuroplasticity—the growth of new neurons and signaling pathways—especially in the hippocampus (the center of learning and memory). IF also lowers inflammation, a major source of cellular dysfunction, throughout the body and encourages autophagy, in which the body clears out dying or damaged cells, helping to deter dementia. The immediate result seems to be a sense of clarity, focus and mental energy.

### Heart

IF has consistently been shown to improve several markers for cardiovascular disease (as well as stroke), including lowering triglycerides and LDL ("bad") cholesterol, which can lead to a thickening of the arteries and arterial obstruction. Inflammation has also been strongly linked to heart disease, and IF is anti-inflammatory.

## Liver

Nonalcoholic fatty liver disease is an obesity-related condition that causes inflammation in the body. It can lead to insulin resistance and is a risk factor for diabetes, heart attacks and even cancer. IF has been shown in studies to reduce fat accumulation in the liver and help prevent fatty liver disease, which afflicts an estimated 25 percent of the U.S. population.

## Waistline

Some of the strongest evidence to date points to IF's efficacy in helping with weight loss, especially dangerous abdominal fat. Once you've been fasting for 12 hours, your body can start burning stored fat instead of recently ingested food; studies show that people on IF lose weight and have a lower body-mass index.

## INFLAMMATION

IF has been shown to lower levels of C-reactive protein, a marker of inflammation in the body. Chronic inflammation has been linked to a long list of disorders, including arthritis, asthma, atherosclerosis, cancer, diabetes and dementia.

## Stomach

Yes, it empties out when you go without food for a while—and there are times when you'll feel hungry on IF. But fasting also changes how your digestive system deals with the "hunger hormones" ghrelin secreted by the stomach lining, it spurs hunger) and leptin (released by fat cells and the stomach, it causes satiety). In a typical calorie-restricted diet, ghrelin soars and leptin drops, so you feel hungry. Fasting seems to do the opposite: Ghrelin may spike at first, then drops lower and stays down, while leptin rises.

## Pancreas

This organ regulates blood sugar by releasing hormones like insulin to bring blood sugar back down to normal after you eat. When you take periodic breaks from eating (even just 14 to 16 hours) the pancreas gets a rest, and insulin levels drop. This process is key to avoiding insulin resistance, a precursor to diabetes in which your cells are exposed to insulin so often that they stop responding to it. The result: blood sugar swings, excess insulin release, weight gain and ultimately diabetes, where blood sugar levels remain high and cause damage to the body.

## Muscles

While calorie-restricted dieting tends to reduce muscle mass, IF instead builds muscle while burning fat for fuel. Part of this is due to growth hormone, more of which is released when you fast. Growth hormone is anabolic (it builds muscle), one reason exogenous forms of it are used in combination with testosterone by bodybuilders.

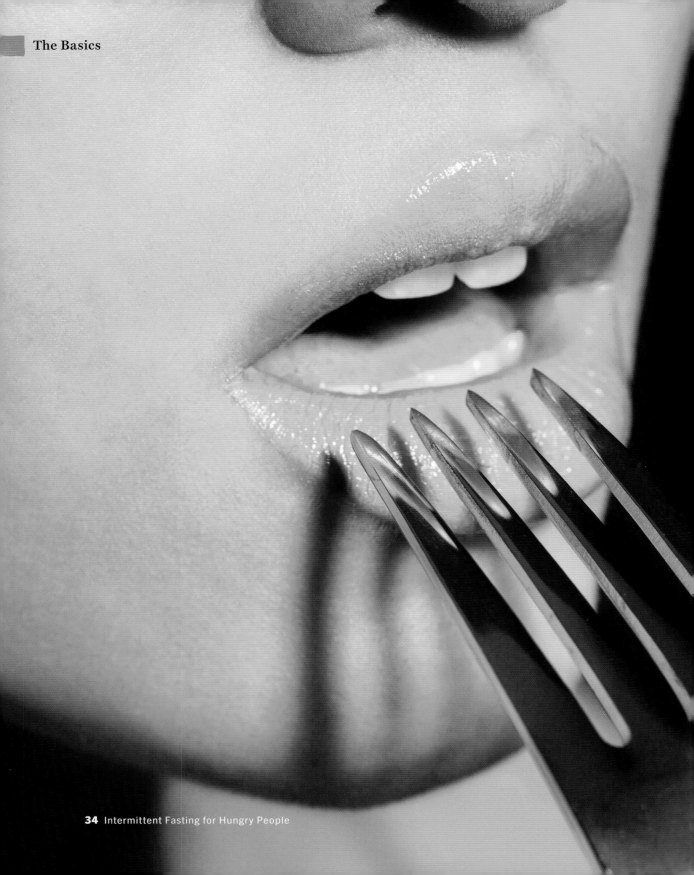

# BUT WON'T I BE
# HUNGRY?

**That's the universal question.
And the answer is: yes and no. Read on
for five key facts about hunger.**

**IT'S SAFE TO** say that as a culture, Americans have developed a fear of hunger. We are deluged with marketing and images that tell us we need that candy bar to stop being "hangry," and that constant fueling with nuts and cheese and between-meal snacks will keep our bodies (and our metabolisms) humming along. We've been warned that getting "too hungry" will make us lose control and binge when we can eat again. Hunger has become an enemy, something to be staved off at all costs, rather than a normal and natural process.

It wasn't always this way—and rates of obesity have never been as high as they are today. "People graze all day long now," says Megan Ramos, co-founder of the Intensive Dietary Management Program. "In the *Leave It to Beaver* days of the late 1950s, the Beav wasn't allowed to eat before

dinner because it would ruin his appetite for the meal. And he wasn't allowed to eat after dinner because that meant he hadn't eaten enough broccoli. That's how our great-grandparents grew up." In those days, hunger was good: It prepared you to sit down and eat a healthy meal, rather than grab a nosh on the run whenever you feel a twinge.

Hunger becomes a bit more fraught, though, when you contemplate going anywhere from 16 hours to a day or more without food. Many people imagine that their hunger will mount to unbearable levels during fasting periods, or that they'll feel weak, shaky or fuzzy-headed. Trust us: You won't. Your body is very well-equipped to handle a little hunger. In fact, going on empty for a time makes it stronger. Here's the (sometimes surprising) news about how hunger works.

## We've Evolved for Hunger

If human beings weren't capable of withstanding periods of food scarcity we wouldn't be here today, explains Peter Bennett, ND, co-author of *7-Day Detox Miracle*. "Our ancestors, living as hunter-gatherers, were fasting at different times, whether they liked it or not," says Bennett. "We're fully wired for it—our physiology is all set up to go for a couple of days without eating. In fact, our bodies kind of like it." That means that rather than feeling weak and confused when hunger pangs start, the body actually powers up, increases metabolism and clears the mind. If it didn't, Homo sapiens would have been too depleted to keep looking for food.

## Expect an Adjustment Period

That said, you may feel a little discomfort when first trying IF. That's because it takes a little time for your body to become fat-adapted—meaning adept at turning to fat stores for fuel. If you've been a snacker for years, your body has been cruising along (and probably gaining weight) on a steady supply of fuel from what you eat. You're able to access stored fat, but you don't need to; over time, those pathways get dusty from disuse. So when you first take away the food-fuel, your body may protest because it has "forgotten" how to get to the fat. The good news, says Ted Naiman, MD, co-author of *The P:E Diet*: "Humans can become fat-adapted, but it takes time and practice. Your body has to do

### Hunger Look-Alikes

Your brain can really fool you when it comes to prompting you to eat. Here are the most common culprits when it comes to "false hunger," according to experts.

**THIRST**
Dehydration often masquerades as hunger. Both can make you feel fatigued, headachy and unfocused, and thirst signals are weak—you tend to not feel specifically dry and parched until you're significantly dehydrated. Sip steadily, whether it's water, coffee or tea, when you're fasting.

**BOREDOM**
Your attention and pep are flagging—and you figure that a hit of "food energy" will perk you up. What you should do first: Distract yourself with another task, whether it's your email inbox or phoning a friend, and see if the pangs fade.

**NEED FOR COMFORT**
It's called "comfort food" for a reason. If you're stressed or depressed, those feelings can be expressed as cravings, especially for carbs because they can raise levels of the "happiness chemical" serotonin. Look for other sources of comfort that don't involve food, like a hot bath, massage or curling up with a favorite book or Netflix show.

**HABIT**
As a society, we have become quite Pavlovian, ruled by external cues when it comes to eating. A study in the *Journal of the American Dietetic Association* asked volunteers to rate their hunger and thirst levels

every hour and also record their eating and drinking schedules for a week. The researchers found that the volunteers seldom ate when they were hungry or drank when they were thirsty. Instead, they simply ate when they normally ate and also drank when they ate. IF changes up these habits so you can become reacquainted with your actual hunger and thirst cues.

**FOOD STIMULI**
Stay out of the kitchen as much as possible. Your body responds automatically, in all kinds of ways, to the sight and smell of food, prompting what feels like hunger—even when you haven't been thinking about food.

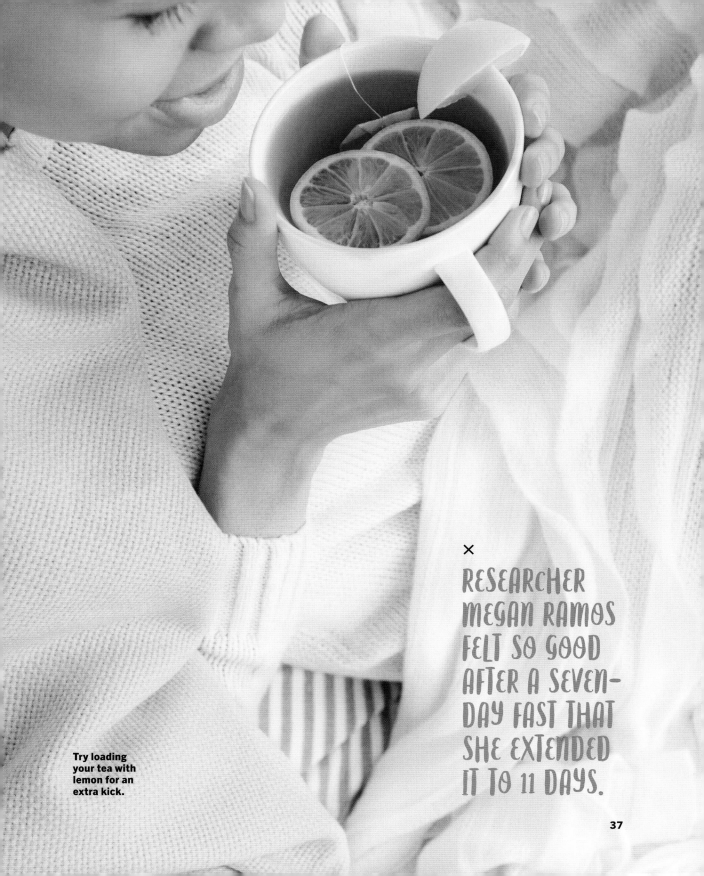

**Try loading your tea with lemon for an extra kick.**

RESEARCHER MEGAN RAMOS FELT SO GOOD AFTER A SEVEN-DAY FAST THAT SHE EXTENDED IT TO 11 DAYS.

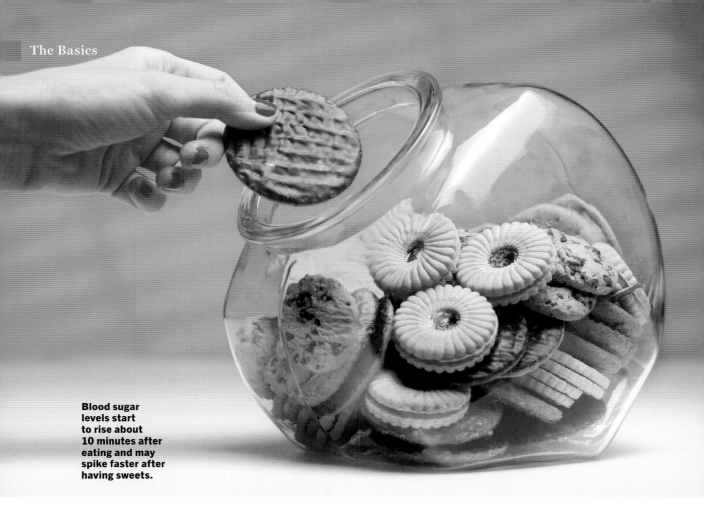

**Blood sugar levels start to rise about 10 minutes after eating and may spike faster after having sweets.**

a number of things to up-regulate your fat-burning pathways—including improving insulin sensitivity, which lowers insulin levels and promotes fat mobilization into free fatty acids from the fat cells." As your body is learning to do this efficiently, it may protest (especially if your insulin is high due to a high-carb diet or insulin resistance). Knowing this is temporary can help you power through.

## Your Hormones Will Help

Hunger and satiety are regulated by several powerful hormones, including appetite-boosting insulin and ghrelin, and satiety-inducing leptin. Over time, they adapt to a fasting regimen. In a study published by the European Journal of Endocrinology, people who fasted for 24 hours (as on a 5:2 or alternate-day program) showed

✕

# OVER TIME, YOUR BODY BECOMES MORE EFFICIENT AT BURNING STORED FAT.

decreasing levels of ghrelin over the fast. "In trials of women fasting for a period of time, we've seen ghrelin go almost to nothing by day three of a fast," says Ramos. You don't need to go on an extended fast to get a hormonal benefit, either. A study in the journal Obesity looked at the 16:8 or time-restricted plan and found that after four days of eating within an eight-hour window, participants had lower ghrelin levels overall and said their hunger felt more "even-keeled." That may be partly because insulin falls during a fast, so you don't have the insulin-fueled blood sugar roller-coaster effect that occurs from constant noshing. The *Obesity* researchers concluded that "meal-timing interventions [like 16:8] facilitate weight loss primarily by decreasing appetite"—the opposite of what you might expect of a fasting plan.

## Hunger Isn't Constant

This surprising truth also has to do with hormones. You may imagine that if you don't feed yourself your hunger will spiral, but that doesn't happen. Think back to a time when you couldn't eat when you were hungry—perhaps you skipped lunch because of a meeting. You probably felt ravenous for a bit…and then forgot about it for a while. Eventually, you started feeling hungry again. That's because ghrelin fluctuates throughout the day due to many factors, including circadian rhythms and habits. For instance, ghrelin is lowest early in the morning, even though you've been fasting while you sleep—one reason many people find that an eating window of, say, noon to 8 p.m. isn't a huge challenge. The *European Journal of Endocrinology* researchers found that in 16:8 fasters, ghrelin spiked at times when the people usually ate. The scientists concluded that "it is the brain that is primarily involved in the regulation of meal initiation."

## Your Own Fat Is Satiating

Here's a funny thing: Just like a fat-loaded steak keeps you satisfied longer than a carb fest, once you are fat-adapted and regularly burning your own fat stores, your hunger level drops. When you oxidize your own fat, it keeps insulin low, because insulin comes into play only when there is sugar in the blood from carbs. "Your fat stores provide your body with a lot of fuel," says Ramos. "So many people, when they do go to eat, find that they're just not that hungry."

## Quick Hunger Fixes
How to surf through the occasional pang? Find relief with these five tactics.

### 1 DRINK UP
Our bodies aren't very good at distinguishing hunger from thirst, so make sure you're well-hydrated. A big glass of water (or sparkling water, with its filling bubbles) can also soothe a grumbling stomach. And studies show that dieters who drank more water lost more weight.

### 2 AVOID CARBS
They are bona fide hunger-boosters because they activate insulin. When you do want to eat a few (healthy, fiber-filled) carbs, try to do it later in the day, advises Ted Naiman, MD. Carbs can "set you up for a blood sugar-and-hunger roller coaster for the rest of the day, contribute to fat storage and sabotage fat burning," he says. Eat them in the evening and you'll sleep through the insulin surge.

### 3 STAY BUSY
Distraction is a powerful tool, so use it. It's one reason 16:8 fasters often break their fast at noon: Once you skip breakfast, you can get caught up in work and avoid hunger until lunch.

### 4 AVOID STIMULI
Food is all around us—but you can push back. Turn out the kitchen light at night, and don't get sucked into social media posts during touch-and-go time—you don't need an Instagram full of culinary masterpieces.

### 5 BE MORE MINDFUL
Hunger is often just a longing for stress relief. Try practicing some mindfulness techniques like deep breathing, yoga or taking a walk outside.

# A LONG
# LEGACY

**What's the furthest thing from a fad diet?
A way of eating that has been around for millennia.
Consider what history tells us about fasting.**

**IT'S HARD TO** imagine a dietary pattern more time-tested than intermittent fasting—although the reasons people followed it in the past ranged much more widely than for weight loss or a longer life. Taking a look at those reasons helps shed light on why fasting is once again having a moment. The difference now? There is so much more in the way of science that backs up its appeal.

## Prehistory

Anthropologists agree that periodic fasts were an inevitable part of early human life, though not by choice. Seasonal shifts, drought, war, insect infestations all brought times of food scarcity, which taught the human body how to survive occasional famines. "We are the product of millennia of feast or famine," says Michael Mosley, MD, author of *The Fast Diet*. "The reason we respond so well to intermittent fasting may be because it mimics, more accurately than three meals a day, the environment in which modern humans were shaped."

## Health and Grace

Eventually, about 12,000 years ago, the invention of agriculture began to make food supplies more reliable. Far from marking the end of fasting,

however, people then began choosing to fast, either for health or in a religious context, raising the question of whether some benefits of fasting had been identified along the way. In the fifth century B.C., Greek physician Hippocrates recommended abstinence from food or drink for patients who exhibited certain symptoms of illness. And some fasted even when healthy. Plato proclaimed, "I fast for greater physical and mental efficiency."

The vast majority of the world's religions incorporate fasting into their rituals, as well. Among ancient civilizations, spiritual fasting was common: The pre-Columbian peoples of Peru fasted after confession, and in many Native American tribes, fasting was practiced before and during vision quests, and during retreats or major ceremonies. To this day, monks (both Christian and Buddhist) regularly fast, and the Buddha himself is said to have come to his enlightenment

✕

## "TO LENGTHEN THY LIFE, LESSEN THY MEALS," SAID BENJAMIN FRANKLIN.

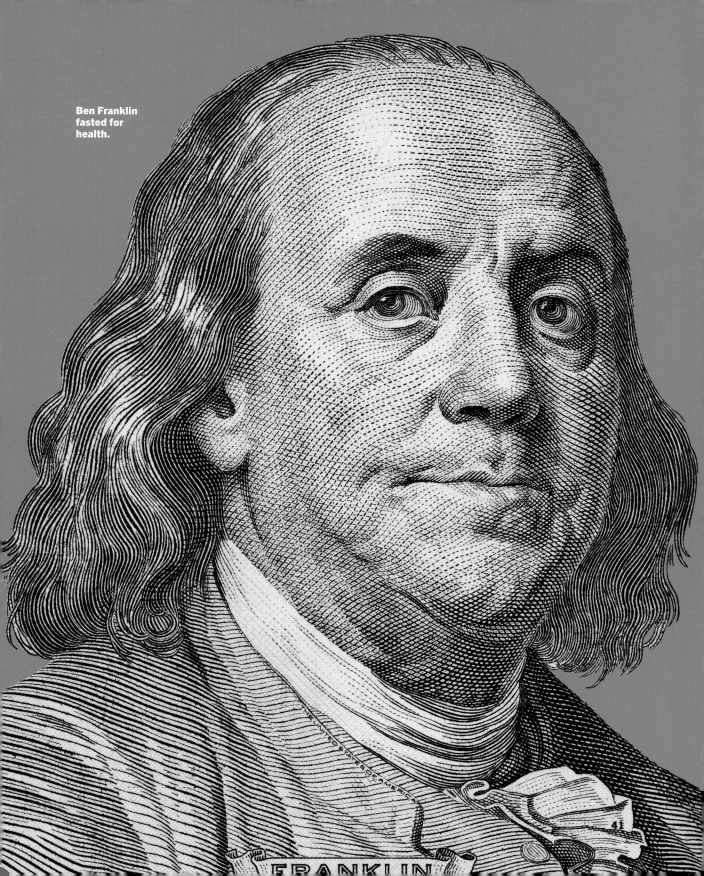

Ben Franklin fasted for health.

41

FRANKLIN

**Fasting led to the Buddha's enlightenment.**

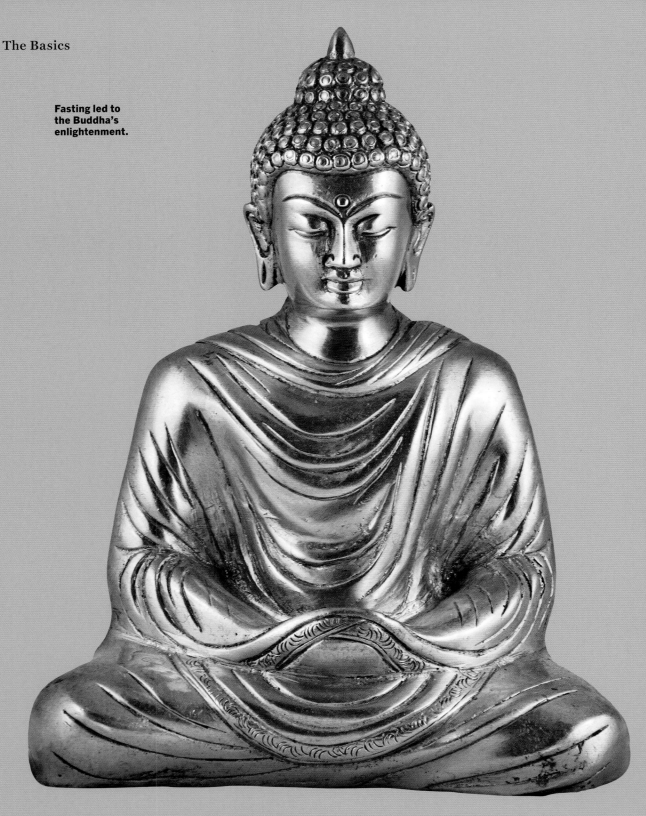

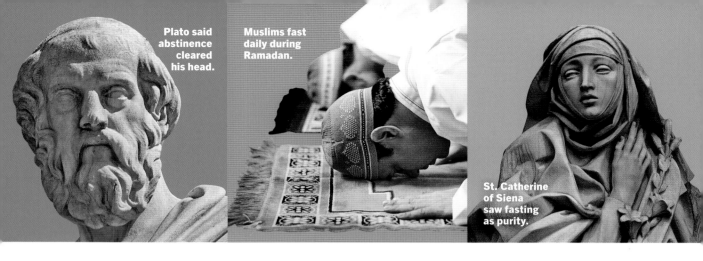

Plato said abstinence cleared his head.

Muslims fast daily during Ramadan.

St. Catherine of Siena saw fasting as purity.

through fasting. One of the most famous religious-fasting practitioners was St. Catherine of Siena, who lived in Tuscany, Italy, in the 14th century and fasted as a way of becoming pure and, she said, having conversations with Jesus.

In modern religious customs, fasting is practiced by Jews (most notably with a full day of fasting on Yom Kippur, the Day of Atonement), Christians (often on Ash Wednesday and Good Friday, as well as avoiding certain foods during Lent), and Muslims (the month of Ramadan, with daily fasting from sunrise to sunset). In all of these, certain ideas are common—enlightenment, spiritual cleansing, visions or feeling closer to God—suggesting that mental clarity has long been seen as one of fasting's effects. That dovetails with new scientific evidence that fasting does indeed show benefits to brain function. The ancients were only a few thousand years ahead of us.

## Spectacle

Fasting took an odd turn in the 19th century, when it became something of a spectator sport. So-called "fasting girls," many of them British, gained fame with claims of living on little to no food, and "fasting artists" actually set up public performances of long-term fasting—memorialized in Franz Kafka's story "The Hunger Artist." One American fasting girl who sparked a news-media frenzy in the 1870s was Molly Fancher, dubbed The Brooklyn Enigma, who claimed to survive for more than a decade on just a few bites of food. Like many of the spiritual fasters, Fancher

✕

# IN THE 19TH CENTURY, PUBLIC FASTING EVENTS HAD THEIR HEYDAY AS ENDURANCE CONTESTS.

claimed to have visions and to have attained a certain purity through avoiding food.

## Longevity

At the same time, various thinkers and writers had signed on to fasting for both optimal health and clear thinking—again echoed in later research, which has turned up many brain and body benefits of intermittent fasting. Ben Franklin proclaimed, "The best of all medicines are resting and fasting," and Mark Twain wrote, "A little starvation can really do more for the average sick man than can the best medicines and the best doctors."

Evidence is emerging that periodic fasting may indeed help deter diseases of aging, like dementia. Several studies of mice genetically altered to develop Alzheimer's disease have found that those fed intermittent fasting diets, compared to those who could eat whenever they wanted, showed better cognitive function, had fewer of the plaques in their brains that can lead to Alzheimer's, and led longer (and healthier) lives.

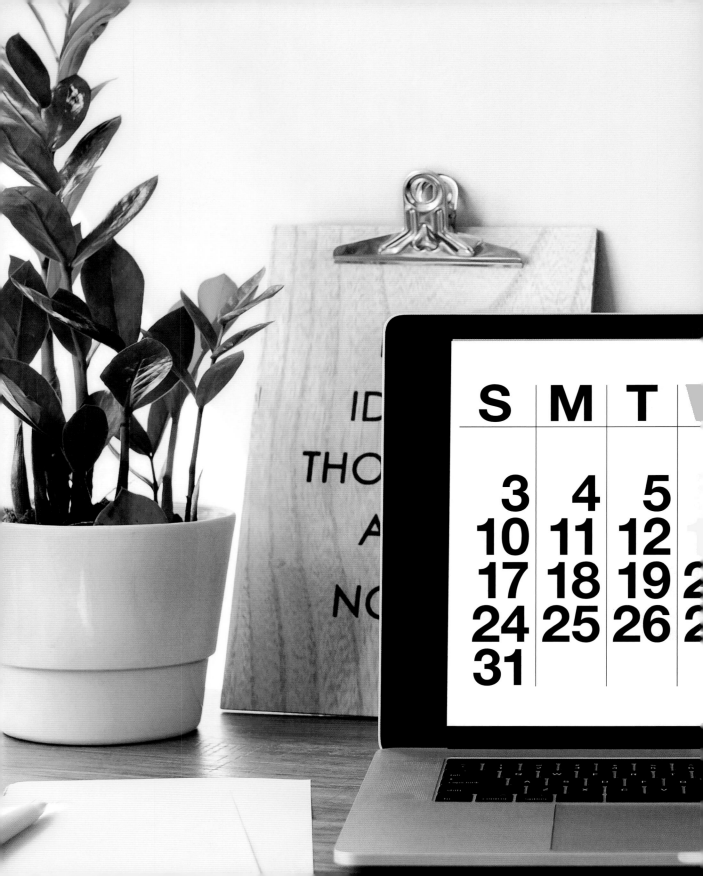

×

# HOW TO GET STARTED

**CHOOSING YOUR
FAST—AND
MAKING IT WORK.**

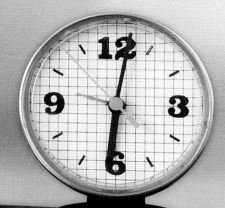

# PICK YOUR
# PLAN

**There are several different approaches
to intermittent fasting—so which one should you try?
A breakdown of the pros and cons of each.**

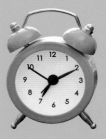

**ONE OF THE** most appealing aspects of IF is
its flexibility. You're rarely hungry for breakfast?
The 16:8 time-restricted plan may be perfect.
Prefer to power through the day and sink into a
big dinner? One meal a day (OMAD) or Warrior
it is. You can also start one plan, see how it goes,
and switch to another if it's not a good fit. The
point to remember, say experts, is that all forms
of IF have benefits. An overview in the *Journal of
the Academy of Nutrition and Dietetics* found that
"almost any intermittent fasting regimen can result
in some weight loss," and "there is little evidence
that intermittent fasting regimens are harmful."

"Go with a schedule that suits you," says
Michael Mosley, MD, author of *The Fast Diet*.
"Whatever you choose, it must be your plan,
your life. Do it with gusto, but be prepared to
experiment within the limits set out by the plan."
Here's what you need to know about each form
of IF before you make your choice.

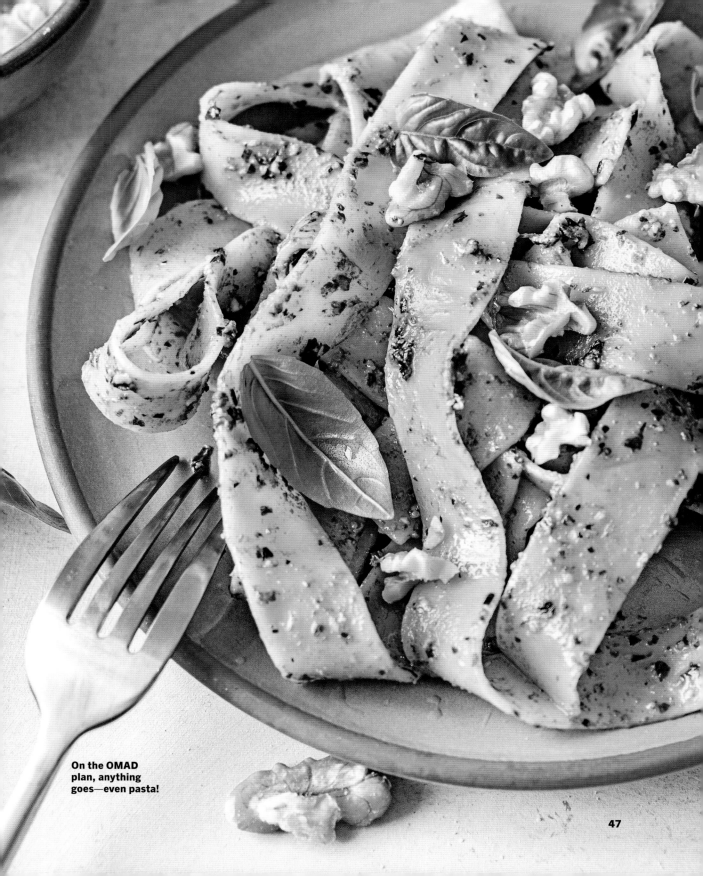

On the OMAD plan, anything goes—even pasta!

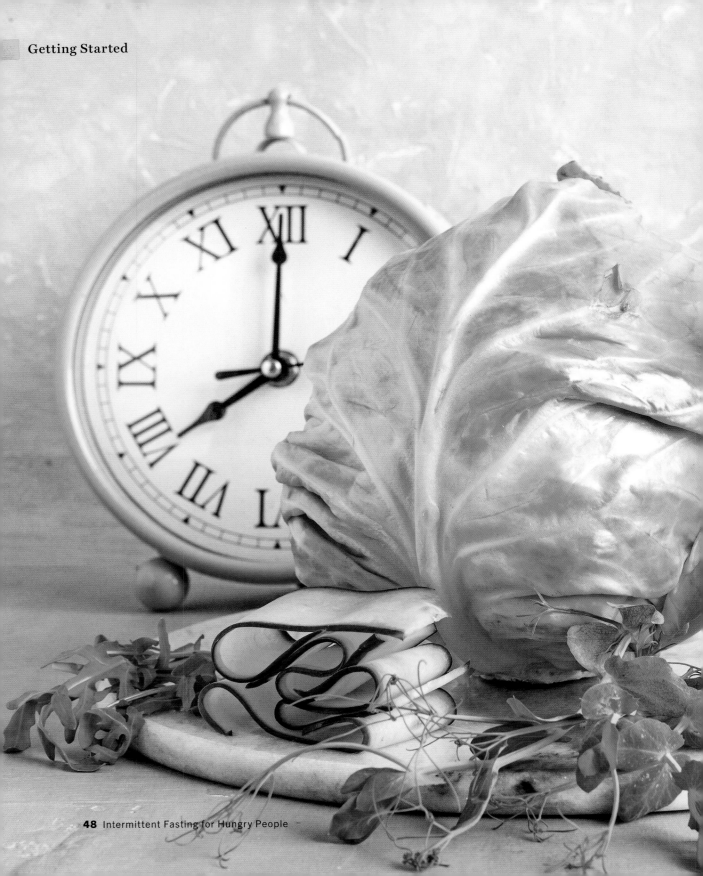

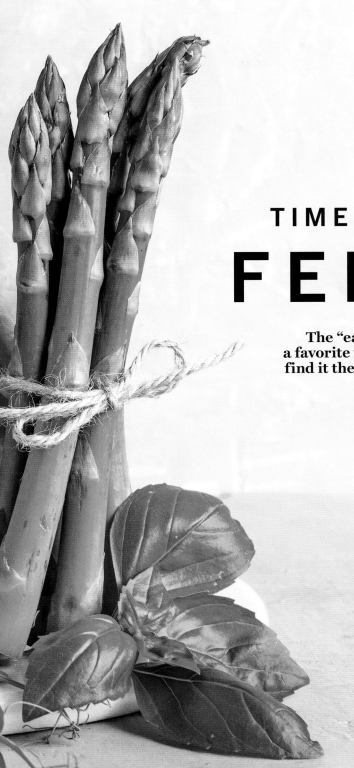

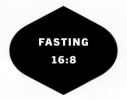

**FASTING 16:8**

## TIME-RESTRICTED
# FEEDING

The "eating window" approach is
a favorite for good reason: Many people
find it the easiest way to fast long term.

**HUGH JACKMAN AND** Jennifer Aniston have sworn by it. Vanessa Hudgens has said it gives her "way more clarity" and makes her feel "more energized and stronger in my workouts." They're talking about the 16:8 plan, a front-runner among fasts and for many people an easy entry point into the intermittent fasting lifestyle. The plan, called variously 16:8 or time-restricted eating, is simple: You just decide where to place your eight-hour eating window, and you eat nothing for the other 16 hours of each day. In practical terms, since you will usually spend seven to eight of those 16 hours sleeping, there are only a few hours of your waking day when you might feel hungry.

Consider, for example, one common format of 16:8: eating between noon and 8 p.m. You'll get up in the morning, and drink water, tea or coffee (though without milk or sugar) to help you wake up and put something in your stomach. If you get up around 7 a.m., that means you'll spend about five waking hours without food. And since most people's circadian rhythms dictate that ghrelin, the primary hunger-inducing hormone, is at its lowest in the morning, many people aren't hungry for at least the first couple of waking hours. Then it's noon, and you can have an omelet or sandwich or salad—any dish you want, depending on whether you're more of a breakfast/brunch or a lunch person. Later, you'll sit down to dinner by 7:30, eat heartily, and then you're done until the next day.

At first glance, this might appear difficult to people who automatically eat breakfast every day (whether they're hungry or not)—but they're in for a surprise. "This may sound drastic and weird, but it's actually been calming," writes beauty blogger Lauryn Evarts Bosstick of her foray into the 16:8 plan. "You don't need to wake up and worry about breakfast, and I think it's lowered my cortisol because I don't need to think about food until lunchtime." Is this plan for you? Read on to find out.

×

## STUDIES SHOW THAT PEOPLE ON 16:8 CONSUME AN AVERAGE OF 300 FEWER CALORIES PER DAY.

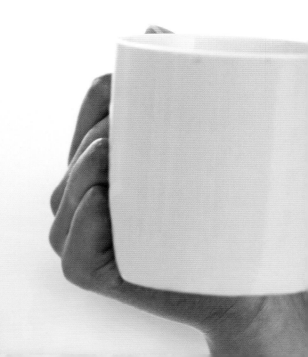

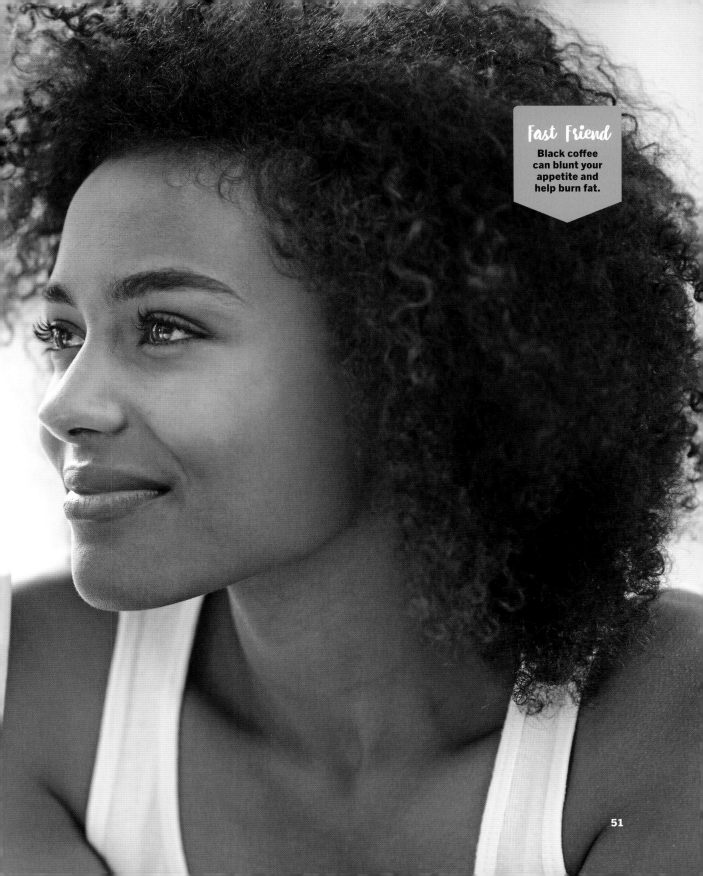

**Fast Friend**
Black coffee can blunt your appetite and help burn fat.

51

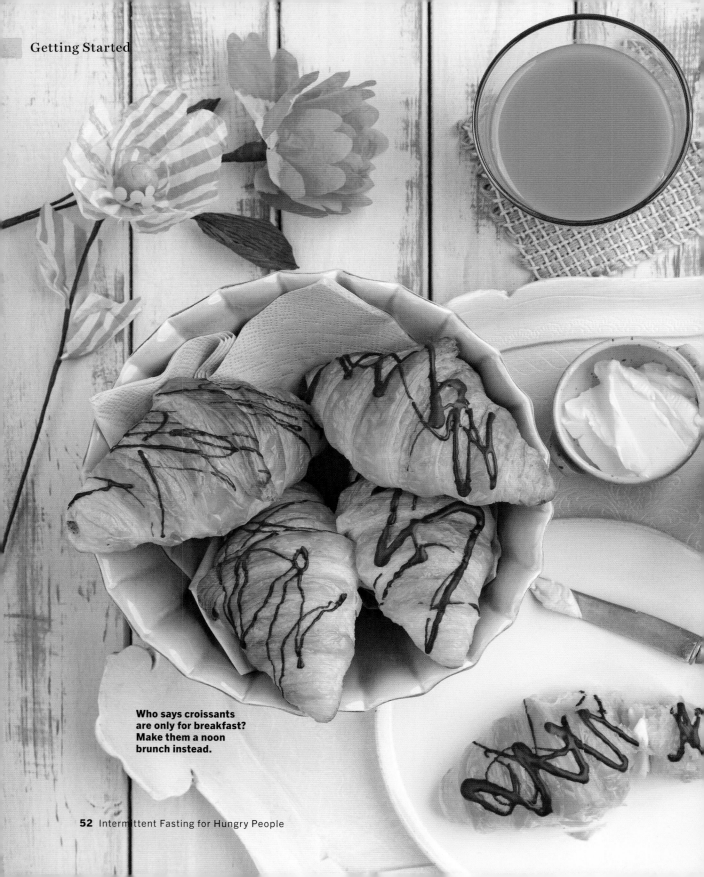

**Who says croissants
are only for breakfast?
Make them a noon
brunch instead.**

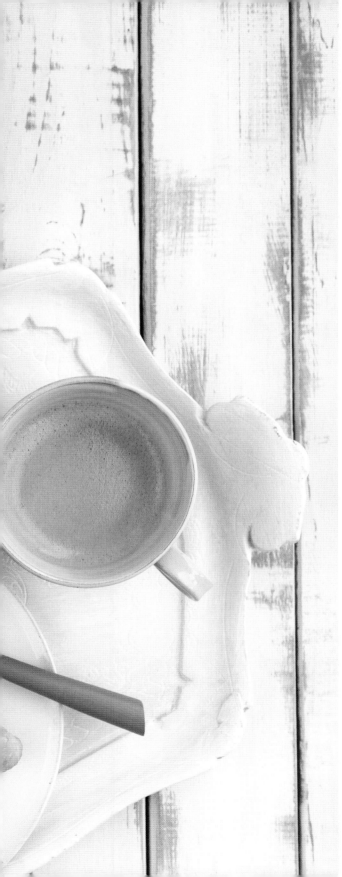

## What the Science Says

Evidence for the effectiveness of 16:8 has been growing in the past few years. A study in the journal *Cell Metabolism* found that time-restricted eating "resulted in weight loss, reduced abdominal fat, lower blood pressure and cholesterol." And, interestingly, the eating window used in the study was 10 hours (14 hours fasting), so it was less rigorous than the 16:8 standard—suggesting that you'll do even better with a smaller window. Study co-author Satchidananda Panda, PhD, commented that participants found the plan "a simple dietary intervention to incorporate," and were easily able to stick to the eating schedule.

That study was a follow-up to research Panda and his team had done in mice and fruit flies. In the mouse study, one group of mice ate all the sugary, fatty foods they wanted on a 24-hour free-feeding schedule. The other group were offered the same foods, but were allowed to eat only during an eight-hour window. The mice with the 24-hour eating window became fat and sick, while the mice in the time-restricted eating window did not. And notably—lest you think those results are due to the 24-hour cohort simply having time to take in more food—both groups ended up consuming the same number of calories. This suggests that simply eating within a smaller window affects how your body deals with the fuel you're loading up on.

In the fruit fly studies, Panda's team found a specific health benefit to time-restricted eating: heart health. The flies who ate in a shorter window

✕

## MORE FASTING HOURS AIDS IN WEIGHT LOSS WHILE IMPROVING SEVERAL HEALTH MARKERS.

had hearts that appeared 20 to 30 percent younger than their age. Panda hypothesized that time-restricted eating helps keep the mitochondria (energy factories) of the heart healthy, reducing oxidative stress over time. As he put it to the American Heart Association after the research was published, "Most of our studies are showing that the effect of time-restricted eating is on multiple organs and on the central nervous system." In other words: The benefits of IF are wide-ranging throughout the body.

## Making It Work

One advantage to 16:8 is that it is especially easy to begin gradually, says Megan Ramos, a clinical researcher and the co-founder of the Intensive Dietary Management Program. "The best place to start is cutting out the snacks. We live such hectic lives that we've lost focus on sitting down and enjoying a meal, so we graze all day. So first, go back to basics and eat only during meals." After you've made some progress with breaking the daytime grazing habit—or the late-evening TV-and-snack habit—Ramos suggests starting to cut out a meal here or there, depending on your goals.

Another way to ease into 16:8 is to begin with a larger eating window and then reduce it over time. For instance, you could start out eating your first meal of the day at 10 a.m. and finishing your dinner at 8 p.m., a 10-hour eating window with a 14-hour fast. As your body adjusts to not snacking outside of those times, you can move it up to 15:9 for a few days or a week, before switching

✕

WANT QUICKER RESULTS? TRY SHORTENING YOUR EATING WINDOW TO SIX HOURS (18:6).

### 16:8
### pros and cons

**PROS**

✳ Zero calorie counting; you should simply aim for a healthy, well-rounded diet during your eating window.

✳ You'll have only a limited number of waking hours when you're fasting, which many find easier to accomplish than a full-day fast.

✳ It conforms easily to your social life—all you have to do is schedule your socializing during your feasting times.

**CONS**

✳ It can be more challenging if you're a morning person.

✳ Weight loss and other health effects may take longer to show themselves than on a more stringent plan.

over to 16:8. At the same time, you can figure out where you want to place your window. If you're a morning person, you may thrive on an earlier schedule, breaking the fast at 10 a.m. and closing the window at 6 p.m. Night owls might want to test-drive a 2 p.m. to 10 p.m. window. The beauty of this plan is that it's effective regardless of when the window opens.

How soon will you see changes? That varies greatly between individuals, says Ramos. The general rule is that after 12 to 16 hours of fasting, your body starts accessing fat stores for energy, "but some people begin burning fat after as little as five hours," she says. If you want to be in that group, Ramos advises, cut down on carbs. "If you're following the standard American diet, which is carb-heavy, you'll store more glycogen, so your body will fuel itself off that for a longer time before turning to body fat." On a low-carb diet you'll have less stored fuel, so your body will become

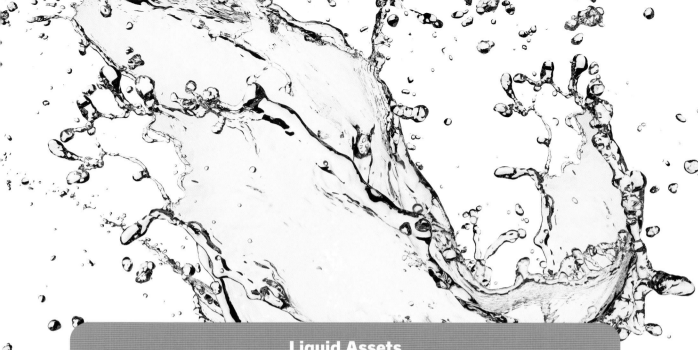

## Liquid Assets

Safe fasting centers on one key guideline: staying hydrated. Not only will you need to drink more water to replace what you normally take in through your food (which is more than you might think!), but zero-calorie liquids are your best friend when it comes to keeping your stomach happy. Here's what you need to know.

### 1 WATER

Go for it! Your muscles, organs and stomach will thank you. If plain $H_2O$ sounds boring, dress it up by infusing it with natural flavors. Put a jug of water in the fridge for between one to 12 hours, adding one of these tasty combos: cucumber slices and mint leaves; lemon and ginger slices; apple slices and a cinnamon stick; or grapefruit slices and a sprig of rosemary. Try seltzer water, too, as the bubbles can be filling.

### 2 TEA

Whether hot or iced, black, green or herbal, tea brings added health benefits. Numerous studies have shown that tea leaves are rich in flavonoids, powerful antioxidants that can lower blood pressure and LDL cholesterol and reduce risk of heart disease. Herbal teas also contain their own array of antioxidants—plus, they help boost the immune and digestive systems.

### 3 COFFEE

After being seen for years as a possible hazard, coffee has emerged as a health star. Studies show it may lower your risk of diabetes, cancer, Alzheimer's disease and depression, and it is considered the biggest source of antioxidants in the Western diet. Its energizing properties also help suppress appetite and break down body fat. Just be sure to drink it black while fasting.

### 4 ALCOHOL

Drinking is allowed when you are practicing intermittent fasting, but there are a couple of caveats to keep in mind: Consuming alcohol has the potential to prompt you to overeat or to make some questionable food choices, and it can also prompt you to continue to sip (and eat!) after your window has officially closed. Plan on pairing any liquor with food, and watch the clock!

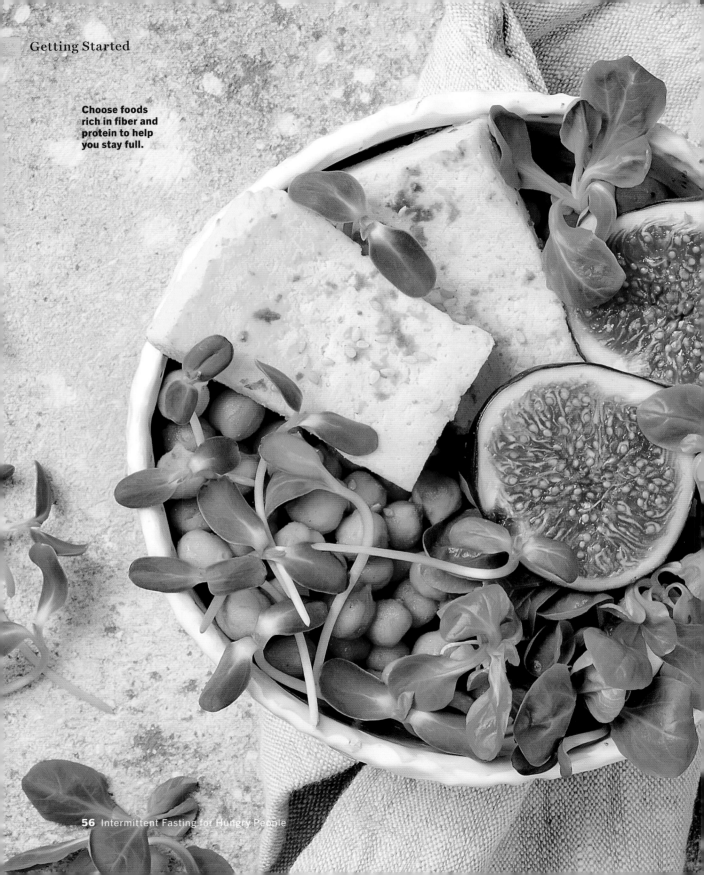

**Choose foods rich in fiber and protein to help you stay full.**

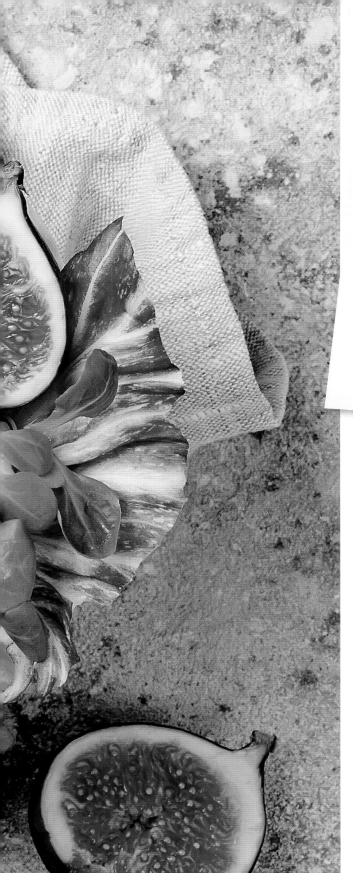

## TRY THIS SAMPLE EIGHT-HOUR MENU

**8:00 A.M.**
Black coffee or tea, and/or seltzer or water with a squeeze of lemon or lime

**NOON–1 P.M.**
Scrambled eggs, whole-wheat toast, bacon or sausage, OR BLT with tomato soup, OR split-pea soup with salad

**6:00–7:30 P.M.**
Chicken breast, Brussels sprouts, brown rice, OR steak, baked potato, salad, OR veggie bowl with rice, mixed vegetables, tofu

"fat-adapted" (i.e., fat-burning) more quickly. The good news is that you can become more efficient at accessing fat stores over time, as your system becomes accustomed to using those fat-burning pathways. (For more on combining a low-carb diet with intermittent fasting, see page 84.)

### The Breakfast Question

Perhaps the most common concern among people doing 16:8 is whether skipping breakfast will be bad for them. For decades, breakfast has been touted as essential—"the most important meal of the day"— by mothers as well as nutritionists

## IF YOU'RE A NIGHT OWL, START YOUR EATING WINDOW AFTER NOON.

and researchers. It was thought that skipping any meal—but especially the first of the day—would lead to overeating later. And various studies seemed to have borne this out, showing that people who regularly skipped meals were more likely to be obese or diabetic.

But these were observational studies, which didn't account for other potential factors: Overweight or obese people, for instance, might skip more meals out of "penance" for overeating at other times. And on the other side of the equation, since eating breakfast was considered a healthy behavior, more fit people who were committed to a healthy lifestyle may have opted for a morning meal, skewing the results.

More recent—and more clinically significant— research has painted a different picture. A meta-analysis of 13 randomized controlled studies published in January 2019 in the journal *BMJ* found that people assigned to eat breakfast actually ate more calories over the course of the day than breakfast skippers. The breakfast fasters didn't overeat later on; in fact, they never compensated for the calories they skipped in the morning. The study also found that people assigned to skip breakfast weighed less than breakfast eaters.

When it comes to the morning-hunger issue, many people find that eating breakfast— especially if it's a typical American (i.e., carb-focused) breakfast—actually spurs more hunger. That's because it can initiate a blood-sugar swing, driving glucose sharply up before a downward dive, prompting your body to crave more carbs. Worried that you'll miss eating your a.m. eggs? Turn your "lunch" into breakfast at noon!

## Three Keys to Success

Experts and experienced time-restricted eaters agree that following these three simple guidelines will make your 16:8 plan easier.

### 1
### LEAN TOWARD LOW-CARB

An important part of IF is dealing with hunger—and eating a higher-fat, lower-carb diet will make hunger less of an issue. Numerous studies show that a high-fat diet is more satiating than a low-carb one. So breaking your fast with a higher-fat (and moderate protein) meal, or ending your day with one, may make the next day easier to handle.

### 2
### DON'T UNDEREAT

Do not try to lower your calorie intake at the same time as doing IF. The whole point of IF is that you can eat "normally" (whatever that means to you) because it's about timing, not calorie-counting. Even more importantly, if you don't eat enough during your eating window, you'll be too hungry to stick to the program.

### 3
### FORGIVE YOURSELF

This is a lifestyle, not a diet. To do 16:8 over the long term, you must accept that every now and then you'll have a day that doesn't fit the plan. It could happen during the holidays, or at a stressful moment, or while traveling and/ or on vacation. Just return to the schedule when you can—and think "marathon" not "sprint."

Deep breathing exercises can create calm and counter cravings.

×

**MINDFULNESS PRACTICES—LIKE FOCUSING ON HOW GOOD YOU FEEL!—CAN HELP GIVE YOU MORE ENERGY ALL DAY LONG.**

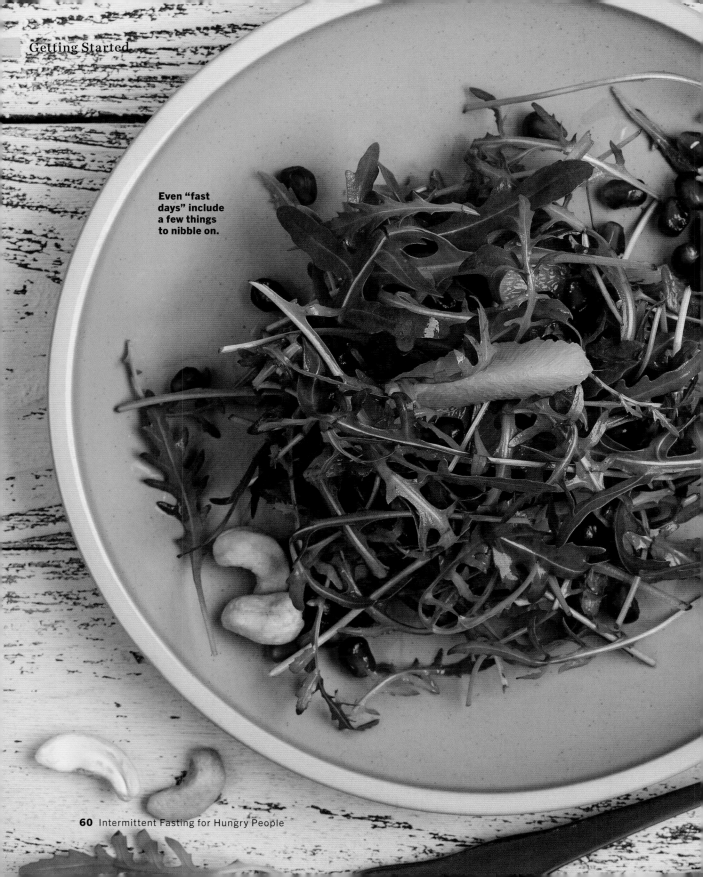

Even "fast days" include a few things to nibble on.

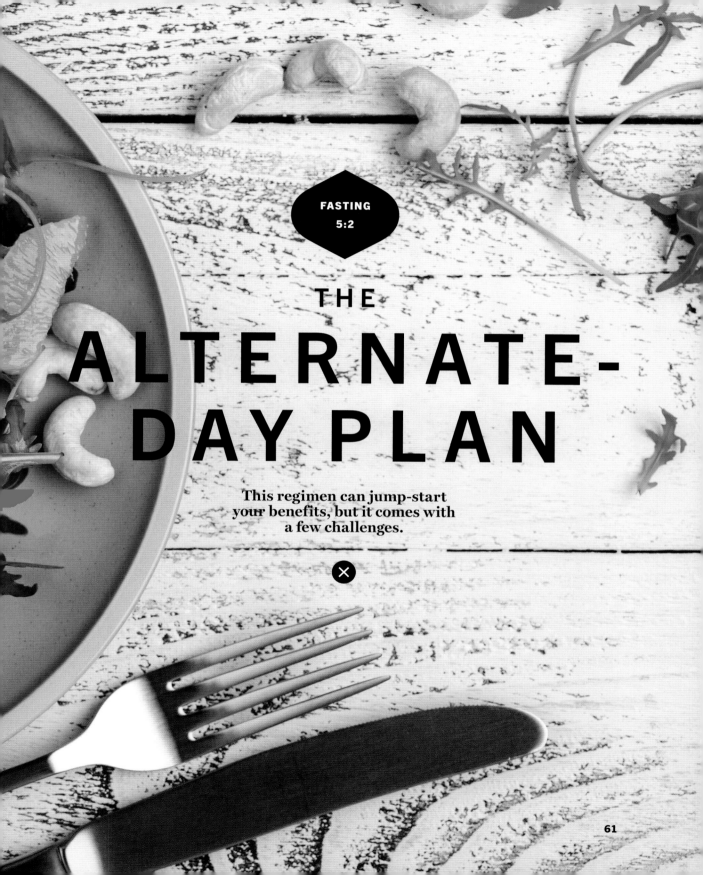

**FASTING
5:2**

# THE
# ALTERNATE-
# DAY PLAN

**This regimen can jump-start
your benefits, but it comes with
a few challenges.**

**IN MANY WAYS,** alternate-day fasting, or ADF, could be considered the OG of fasting. Long before intermittent fasting became the dieting flavor of the year, scientists were examining the health effects of going without food—or with very little food—for a day at a time. It started a century ago, when researchers began studying the health impact in laboratory animals of reducing overall food intake by 30 to 40 percent, and found that they lived longer and had a reduced incidence of cancer. Then in the 1940s, a new paradigm was introduced: Rather than lowering food intake 24/7, lab rats were made to fast on alternate days and offered regular chow on the feast days. According to a study in the journal *Age*, researchers found that, just like the chronically underfed rats in previous studies, the ADF rats lived considerably longer and had a much lower incidence of cancer.

The real breakthrough, though, came decades later. Scientists had assumed that the benefits of ADF were simply due to the rats eating less, making them similar to the rats who had overall reduced food intake. They were astonished to find that instead, those rats managed to cram as many calories into their feasting days as the control-group rats who could eat whenever they wanted. The upshot: The benefits of ADF were not due to eating less food into perpetuity, but to some other mechanism—or

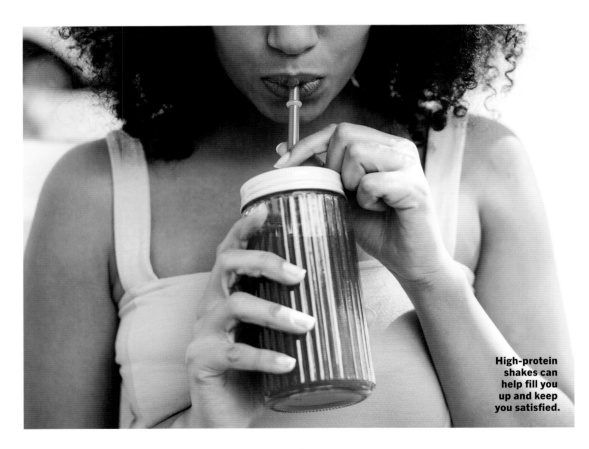

**High-protein shakes can help fill you up and keep you satisfied.**

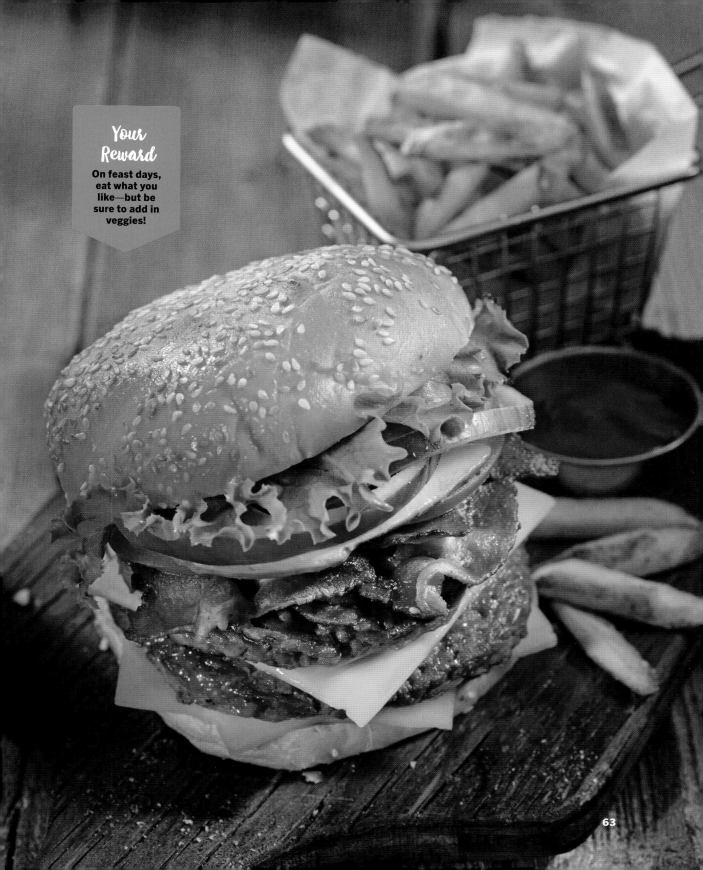

**Your Reward**

On feast days, eat what you like—but be sure to add in veggies!

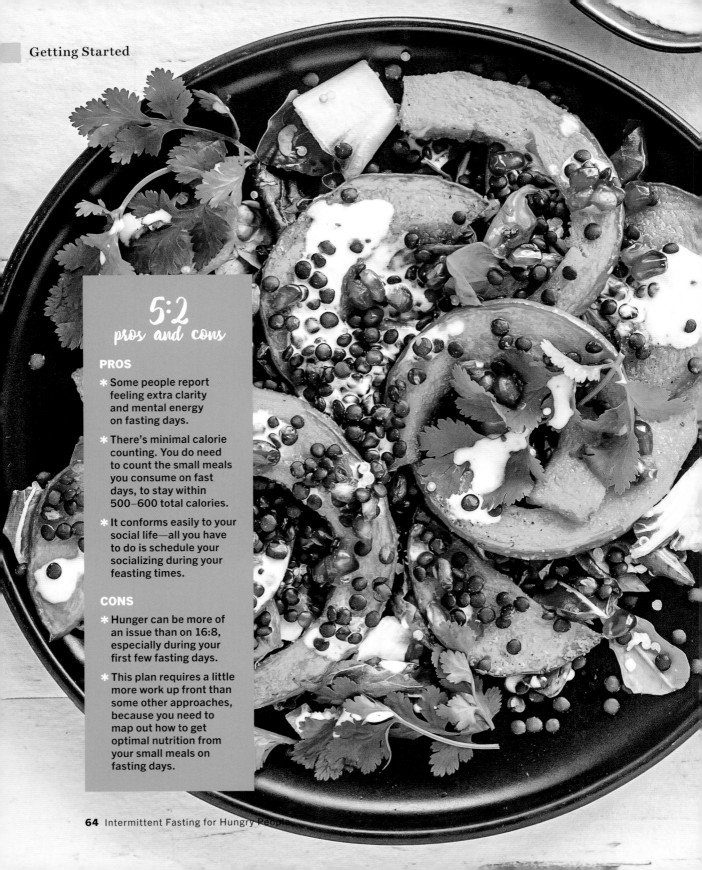

# 5:2
## pros and cons

### PROS

* Some people report feeling extra clarity and mental energy on fasting days.

* There's minimal calorie counting. You do need to count the small meals you consume on fast days, to stay within 500–600 total calories.

* It conforms easily to your social life—all you have to do is schedule your socializing during your feasting times.

### CONS

* Hunger can be more of an issue than on 16:8, especially during your first few fasting days.

* This plan requires a little more work up front than some other approaches, because you need to map out how to get optimal nutrition from your small meals on fasting days.

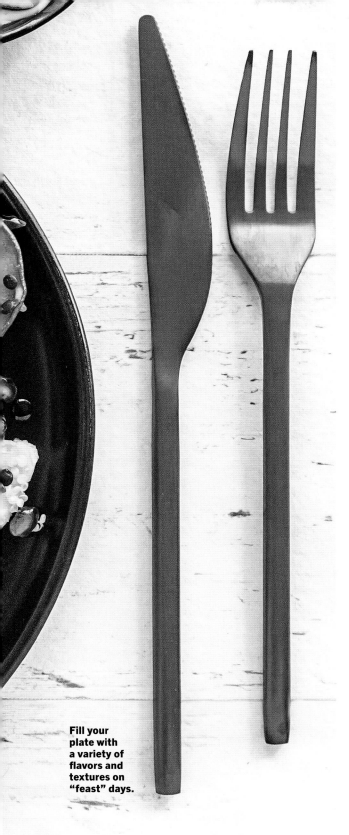

**Fill your plate with a variety of flavors and textures on "feast" days.**

×

# "IF YOU GET HEADACHES ON FAST DAYS, DRINK MORE WATER," ADVISES RESEARCHER KRISTA VARADY, PHD.

multiple mechanisms. Since then, some of these have come into focus: Fasting's numerous perks appear to be tied to all kinds of molecular changes, including an increase in growth hormone, regulation of glucose and insulin levels, and a process called hormesis, in which a certain level of cellular stress kicks all kinds of damage-repair processes into gear.

In other words, if you want to try this form of IF, you don't need to consign yourself to a lifetime of undereating in order to get healthier, lose weight and live longer. You simply need to rearrange your eating times, and during your feast times, you can graze to your heart's content.

Of course, studies in rats are not conclusive—they can hint at results and pathways, but they're not the final word on human health. But in the past few years, human clinical trials have supported the original hypothesis. For instance, a review of human studies in the *Journal of the Academy of Nutrition and Dietetics* found that "alternate-day fasting appears to result in weight loss as well as reductions in glucose and insulin concentrations." And a study in the journal *Cell Metabolism* randomized participants into two groups, one doing ADF and the other not, for four weeks. They found that ADF led to fat loss, especially in the abdominal region, with an improved fat-to-lean ratio—meaning more muscle mass was retained—as well as reduced blood pressure and a reduction in the overall cardiac risk score.

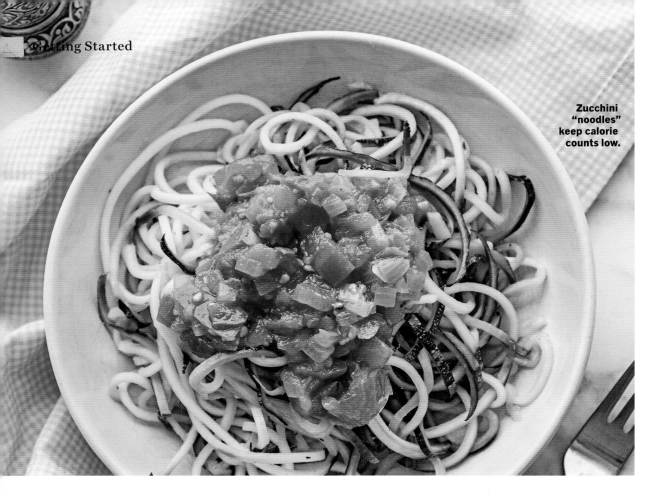

**Zucchini "noodles" keep calorie counts low.**

Perhaps the most intriguing result in the *Cell Metabolism* study was the view it offered of ADF's effects on all kinds of key health markers. The researchers found that ADF increased levels of an important ketone, B-hydroxybutyrate or BHB, even on nonfasting days. BHB functions as an alternate fuel, and is thought to be a main source of the health benefits of a keto diet, especially brain health. The study also showed that on fasting days there was a decrease in a pro-aging amino acid called methionine—a hint at why ADF may have anti-aging properties. At the same time, there were reduced levels of sICAM-1, an age-associated inflammatory marker, as well as LDL cholesterol (the bad kind). The same study also separately followed 30 people who practiced

ADF for six months, and found that there were no negative side effects compared to a control group. In other words, ADF was shown to be both safe and effective.

## The 5:2 Variation

Well fine, you may be thinking, but how hard is this to carry out? The answer to that depends on who you ask—and ADF may not be for everyone. "When we first started studying alternate-day fasting, we wondered whether it was realistic to ask people to drop down to only 500 calories a day, every other day," says Krista Varady, PhD, a professor of nutrition at the University of Illinois at Chicago, and author of *The Every Other Day Diet*. "But we found that many people actually could stick to the diet for two months, and lost between 10 and 30 pounds." On the other hand,

# A Visual Guide to Your 5:2 Days

You may be surprised at what you can eat while still staying between 500 and 600 calories. It's a matter of two things: learning your calorie counts, and going for big flavor. Use this mix-and-match chart to plan two meals for your fast days—or combine them into one larger meal.

## MEAL NO. 1

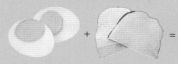 = **155** CALS.

Boiled egg
**75 CALS.**

3 oz. ham
**80 CALS.**

 +  = **135** CALS.

4 ounces 2% fat cottage cheese
**105 CALS.**

1 fig
**30 CALS.**

 +  = **137** CALS.

6 ounces full-fat yogurt
**105 CALS.**

½ cup raspberries
**32 CALS.**

### SWAPS

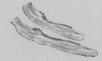

2 slices bacon
**90 CALS.**

½ pear
**40 CALS.**

## MEAL NO. 2

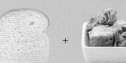 +  +  = **209** CALS.

1 slice light bread
**45 CALS.**

6.5 ounces tuna
**144 CALS.**

1 teaspoon light mayo
**20 CALS.**

 +  +  = **131** CALS.

2 cups zucchini noodles
**40 CALS.**

½ cup tomato sauce
**70 CALS.**

1 tablespoon Parmesan
**21 CALS.**

 +  +  = **208** CALS.

4 ounces boneless chicken breast
**136 CALS.**

1 teaspoon olive oil
**36 CALS.**

3 broccoli spears
**36 CALS.**

### SWAPS

1 cup chicken noodle soup
**70 CALS.**

1 cup split-pea soup
**150 CALS.**

1 tomato
**24 CALS.**

she adds, "People who are frequent snackers and are used to eating something every two to three hours may not do as well with it." And the first 10 days, Varady cautions, "are pretty tough. It can be hard to adjust to that up-down pattern of eating." Once you've weathered five fasting days, though, your body adapts to the rhythm of fast-and-feast.

One way to make the program a little easier, says Varady, is to do a modification of ADF called the 5:2 plan, in which you have only two fasting days a week, eating normally on the remaining five days. "Most people choose to fast on Monday and Wednesday or Thursday, because having a fast day on the weekend is more difficult," Varady says. As for when and how to consume those 500 to 600 calories, it's up to you: Some people choose to put them all in one meal; others create two meals (say, a breakfast/brunch and a dinner); or you can try eating three small meals to mimic a normal day.

Varady has also studied which patterns tend to work best, instructing participants to eat either one meal at lunchtime, one at dinnertime, or small meals throughout the day. "The timing didn't influence weight loss, but the people in the dinnertime group found it much easier to do. We had lots of complaints about feasibility in the lunchtime group, and people found the small meals pretty brutal—if you're hungry and can eat only 100 calories, it can be hard. And most social things happen at night or around dinnertime." That said, if you're a morning person, go for it. And if you decide to try two meals on your fasting day, see page 67 for ideas that can help you make the most of your calorie allotment.

# FASTING DOESN'T MEAN NO FOOD—SMALL MEALS CAN HELP TIDE YOU OVER.

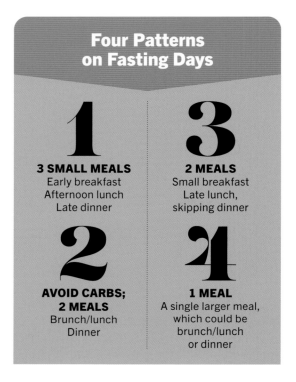

## Four Patterns on Fasting Days

### 1
**3 SMALL MEALS**
Early breakfast
Afternoon lunch
Late dinner

### 3
**2 MEALS**
Small breakfast
Late lunch,
skipping dinner

### 2
**AVOID CARBS; 2 MEALS**
Brunch/lunch
Dinner

### 4
**1 MEAL**
A single larger meal,
which could be
brunch/lunch
or dinner

## What to Eat

One important point about both 5:2 and ADF: Your menu on fasting days counts for a lot. "Try to consume a fair amount of protein on fast days, shooting for about 50 grams," Varady advises. "That's about 40 percent of your calories. You could have a salad with a lot of meat or beans on it, or a high-protein shake. That will help stave off hunger." Your reward is feast day, where anything goes—within reason.

On your feast days, you should avoid processed foods as much as possible and focus on consuming fresh, whole foods. But the beauty of ADF is that you can eat like you're not on a "diet," says Varady. "I had wondered whether people would binge on their feast days, but our studies of hundreds of people have shown that most eat only about 10 percent more than usual. And they told us they felt fuller faster, and could control their appetite better."

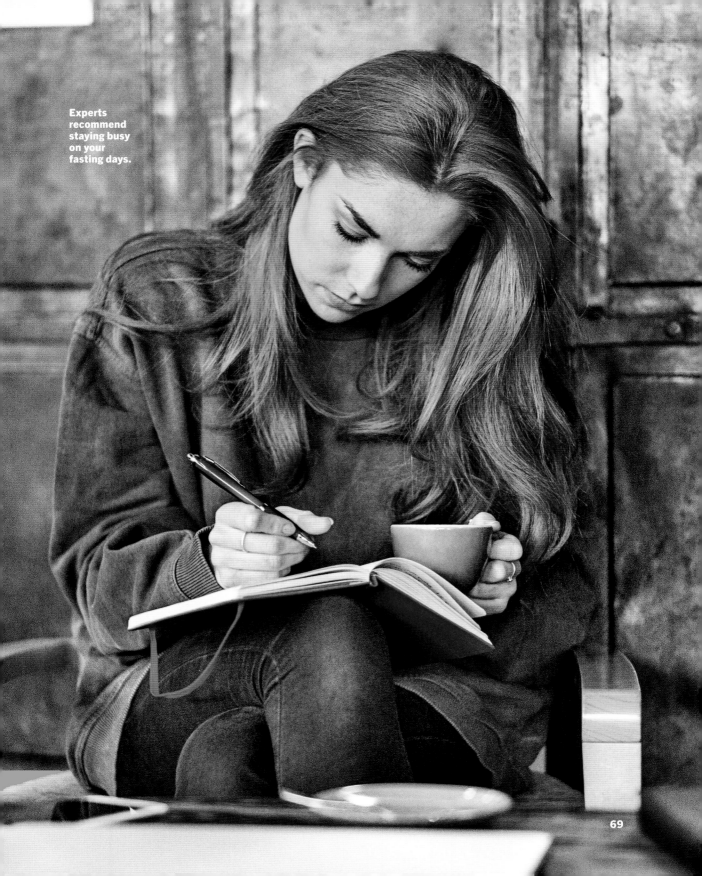

Experts recommend staying busy on your fasting days.

69

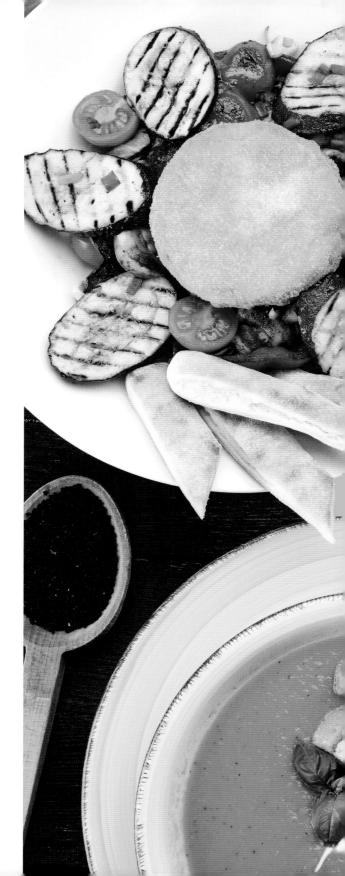

**FASTING OMAD OR WARRIOR**

# ONE MEAL A DAY

### Called OMAD or Warrior for short, this plan with prehistoric roots puts all the emphasis on a delicious dinner.

**TALK ABOUT COUNTERINTUITIVE:** Not only does OMAD go against recent dietary advice to not go too long between meals, it also breaks the "don't eat too much at night" rule. And yet, its proponents claim that it effectively mimics the way our bodies evolved to thrive in ancient times. Hunter-gatherers are thought to have eaten sparingly during the day while they sought food, and then feasted at night. So far, science is showing that OMAD fans may be right, as early research shows that the plan has benefits similar to other forms of intermittent fasting—making

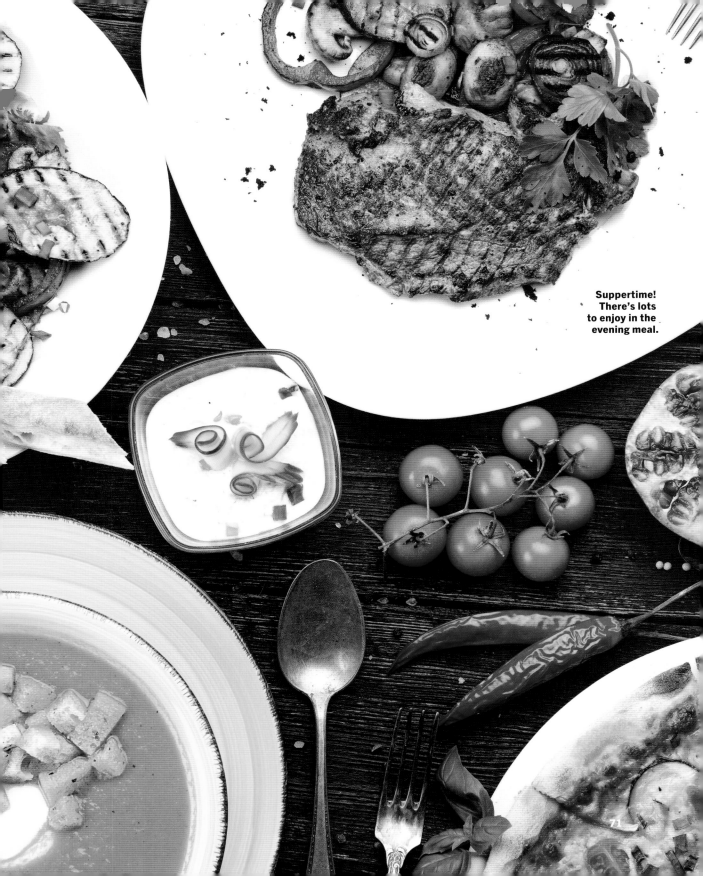

**Suppertime!
There's lots
to enjoy in the
evening meal.**

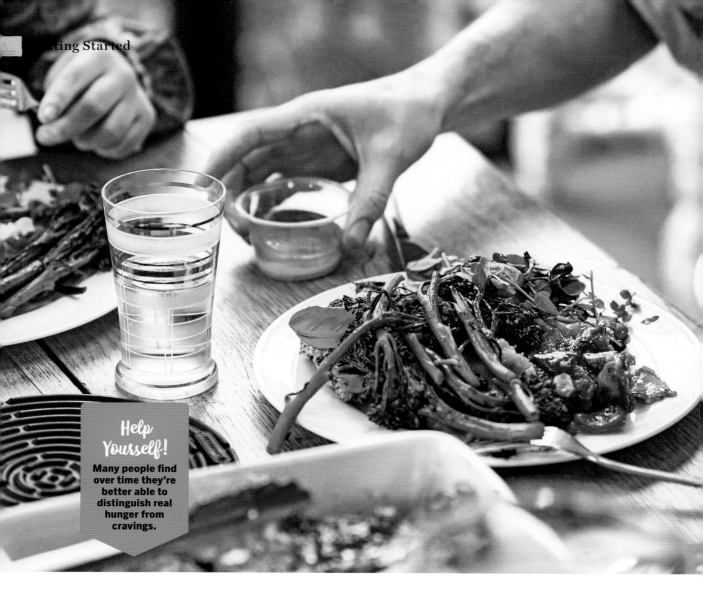

**Help Yourself!**

Many people find over time they're better able to distinguish real hunger from cravings.

it a good choice for people who prefer to power through the day on fumes and then indulge in the evening.

Some of the first studies of OMAD were observational and focused on groups of people who have been practicing this form of fasting for millennia: Muslims who celebrate Ramadan for one month a year. That religious observance calls for fasting from sunrise to sundown, followed by nightly feasts. A meta-analysis in the journal *Public Health Nutrition* in 2012 found statistically significant weight loss in nearly two-thirds of

studies of Ramadan fasters. The following year, the *Journal of Religion and Health* published another meta-analysis, this one looking at biomarkers of health and disease in Ramadan fasters. It found that after the month of Ramadan, fasters had lower levels of LDL cholesterol and blood-glucose levels, and in women, HDL cholesterol (the good kind) increased significantly. Other studies have shown that Ramadan fasts are associated with lower levels of inflammatory markers such as C-reactive protein (CRP) and interleukin 6 (IL-6).

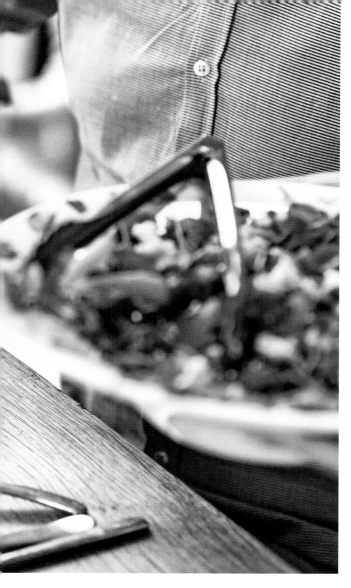

×

# NIGHT OWLS ENJOY THE ABILITY TO KICK BACK WITH A SUPER-SATISFYING WARRIOR-STYLE DINNER.

## OMAD or Warrior?

These two names for one meal a day actually refer to two slightly different ways of going about timing your eating. One meal a day is, in effect, a kind of supercharged 16:8—in which the eating window is made considerably shorter than eight hours—and OMAD and Warrior are on a sliding scale. The Warrior plan is essentially a four-hour eating window (20:4), while OMAD narrows that window down to just one hour (23:1).

The Warrior plan was popularized in 2001 by Ori Hofmekler, author of *The Warrior Diet* and a former member of the Israeli Special Forces who transitioned into the field of fitness and nutrition, and it is as much a philosophy as an eating regimen. When he introduced the plan, he wrote, "Many people today have an irrational—almost phobic—fear of hunger." Hofmekler sees the Warrior approach as a way to harness hunger for good: "Hunger will trigger the active part of the survival instinct—that which makes you more alert, ambitious, competitive and creative."

Interestingly, this dovetails with research that shows IF in general tends to increase energy and mental clarity rather than sluggishness. And because Warrior is based on prehistoric eating patterns, many people pair it with a paleo food plan, avoiding processed and farmed foods and eating only whole, preagricultural foods: fish, meat, fruits, vegetables, nuts and seeds.

More recently, a randomized, controlled trial in healthy, normal-weight adults put these observations to the test. First, the test group ate three meals per day for a period of eight weeks. Then, after a break, the same group ate one meal a day for another eight weeks. The result was "a significant modification of body composition, including reductions in fat mass." Other studies looking at OMAD are still ongoing. But does it make sense to cluster almost all your calorie intake at the end of the day? Read on to get the full OMAD story.

OMAD, on the other hand, is more the product of modern thinking about IF, based on the fact that the longer you extend your fast, the more time you give your body to burn fat. Most people switch from stored glycogen to stored fat after about 12 hours of fasting, so if you go another eight to 11 hours, you'll torch even more.

Another reason why OMAD and Warrior work, though, may be simply that there's only so much food anyone can eat at one time, whether it's an hour or four hours, says Krista Varady, PhD, a professor of nutrition at the University of Illinois at Chicago, who has studied intermittent fasting extensively. Varady conducted a study where participants were required to eat between 3 p.m. and 7 p.m. every day for two months. The average weight loss was about 10 pounds, along with reductions in blood pressure, insulin, insulin resistance and oxidative stress.

Varady found that researchers practically had to "force-feed" participants to squeeze enough food into their window—and they still lost weight.

"Eating 2,000 calories, or even 1,500 calories, in one sitting is kind of tough for people," Varady says. Considering that the average American takes in more than 3,600 calories a day, according to data from the United Nations (up 24 percent since 1961), going down even to 2,000 is, for many people, a big reduction in energy intake.

## Those P.M. Calories

One stumbling block for some dieters, and even for some experts, is the long-touted advice that nighttime calories are bad news—hence the expression, "Breakfast like a king, lunch like a prince, and dinner like a pauper." Some studies have shown that eating late in the day is associated with higher body weights. But many researchers argue that an association is not necessarily a cause. If someone is noshing on late-night snacks on top of a full day of eating, that's a far different calorie load than someone who eats only one meal, which just happens to occur at the end of the day.

## What and When to Eat: One Meal a Day

### With only one meal a day, the focus is on the quality of your diet. Here's how to eat well.

Some people doing OMAD/Warrior interpret the "fasting" period to mean that you can nibble a bit—usually just a few raw veggies to keep calories very minimal. Staying hydrated is also essential, so fill up on lots of water or seltzer, along with black coffee or tea.

When it comes time for your big evening meal, it's key that your choices are well-balanced nutritionally and include plenty of satiating fats and protein with minimal or no processed foods.

After all, you're packing all your nutrients, antioxidants, vitamins and minerals into that one meal! Fill your plate with a variety of healthy options, including components like these:

**HEALTHY FATS** Try olive oil, avocado oil and coconut oil.

**WHOLE GRAINS** Opt for quinoa, brown rice and oats.

**FRUITS** Choose berries, papaya, mango and oranges.

**MEAT, POULTRY AND FISH** Look for wild-caught fish and organic, pasture-raised meat and poultry.

**LEAFY GREENS** Load up on superfoods like kale, collards, spinach and chard.

**OTHER COLORFUL VEGGIES** Some best bets include white and sweet potatoes, beets, carrots, broccoli, asparagus, Brussels sprouts, bell peppers, butternut squash and zucchini.

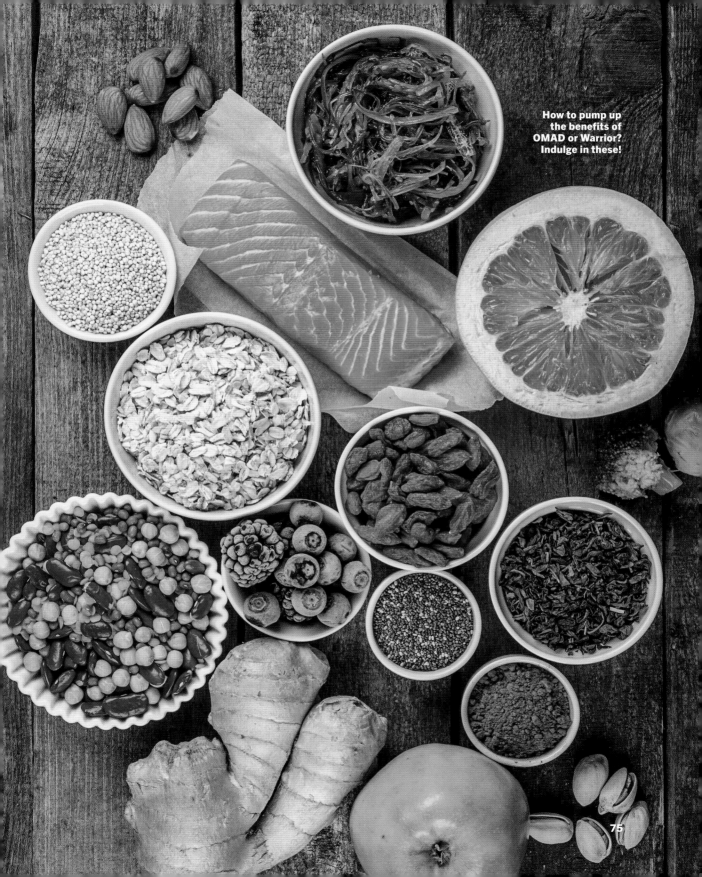

How to pump up
the benefits of
**OMAD** or **Warrior**?
Indulge in these!

75

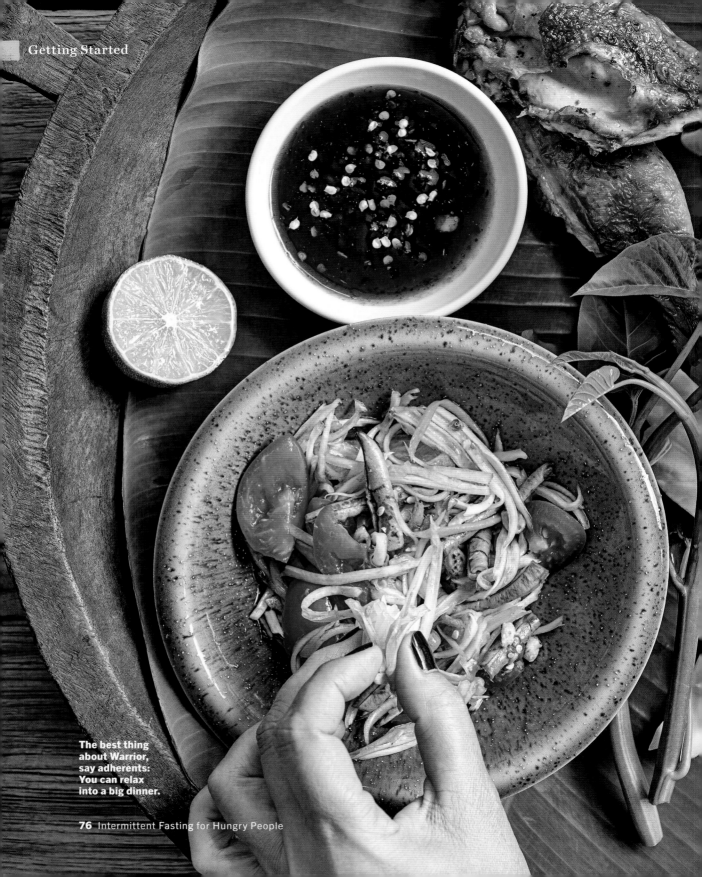

The best thing about Warrior, say adherents: You can relax into a big dinner.

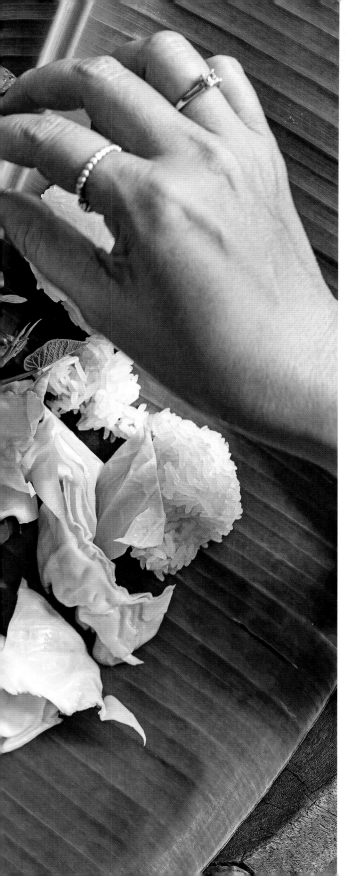

"The longer you stay in the fasted state, the more metabolic practice you will get at burning stored body fat," explains Ted Naiman, MD, co-author of *The P:E Diet*. "If you can maintain this intermittent fast for 20 hours or more, you'll reach a high rate of lipolysis—the breakdown of stored body fat into free fatty acids available for burning in the cells—and fat oxidation." Fasting early in the day and eating later may also maximize the body's natural shifts between sympathetic ("fight-or-flight") and parasympathetic ("rest-and-digest") nervous-system tones. This means you have higher alertness from sympathetic tone while undereating during the day, and higher parasympathetic resting tone in the evening, during the fed state.

# OMAD/WARRIOR
## pros and cons

### PROS

* Mornings (and a.m. workouts) may be easier because you're still fueled from your big dinner.

* Less planning! Some people say they feel freed from cooking, or buying, breakfast and lunch, and the regimen calls for a very satisfying meal at the end of the day.

* That one big meal tends to be extra-enjoyable, Warriors report, after the daylong fast.

### CONS

* Hunger! Tolerance for this plan is highly individual: Some people cruise through their day while others may struggle.

* Temptation: If your life, or workday, calls for being around food a lot—say you're feeding your kids breakfast and lunch, or doing business over lunch with clients— OMAD may be more of a challenge.

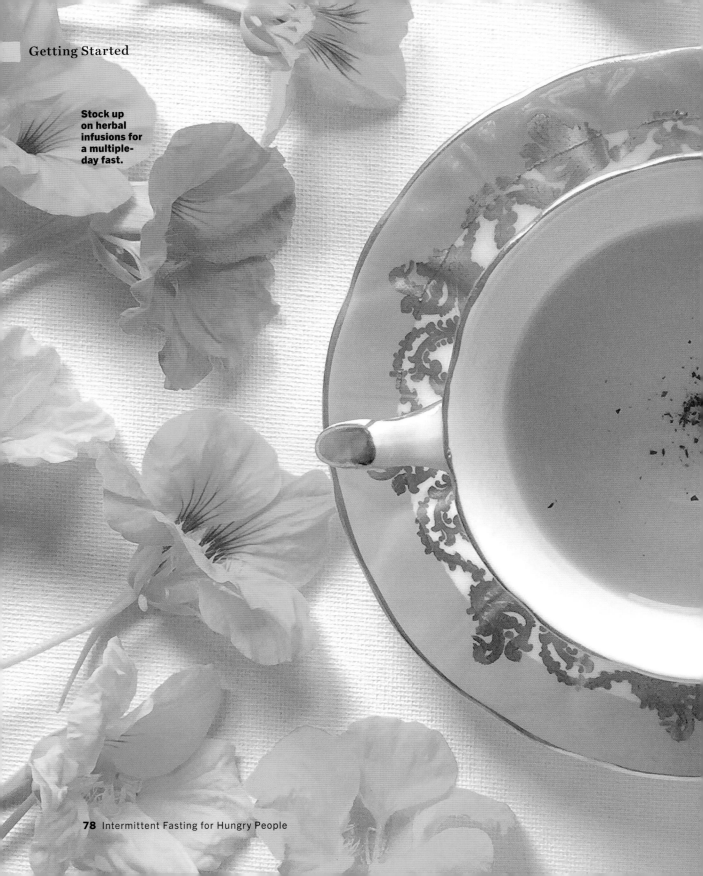

**Stock up
on herbal
infusions for
a multiple-
day fast.**

# LONGER FASTS

**Holding out for more than
a day brings accelerated results.
Here's how to do it safely.**

**GOING MORE THAN** a day without food? At first glance, many people might find that concept alarming. The evidence keeps piling up, however, that not only does an extended fast supercharge the benefits—including faster weight loss and more profound changes to health markers like blood pressure and growth-hormone levels—but it also may not be as hard to accomplish as you might think.

Fasts that last longer than 24 hours were once a fringe concept, or something linked to religious practices (think of the 40 days of fasting detailed in the Bible's Temptation of Christ). But in these days of soaring rates of metabolic diseases like diabetes and obesity, extended fasts are becoming an extremely useful (and doable) option, says Megan Ramos, co-founder of the Intensive Dietary Management Program. "It's a more therapeutic level of fasting," Ramos says. She cites clients who have, as a result of extended fasts, seen reversals of serious ailments, including metabolic syndrome, a cluster of conditions (high blood pressure, high blood sugar, excess abdominal fat and high cholesterol) that together raise your risk of heart disease, stroke and Type 2 diabetes.

That experience is borne out in studies. One published in 2019 in *PLOS ONE* followed more than 1,400 subjects over one year; they participated in a program consisting of fasting periods of between four and 21 days (in this study, "fasting" meant a daily calorie

✕

## A 2019 STUDY FOUND THAT A 58-HOUR FAST SIGNIFICANTLY RAMPED UP HUMAN METABOLISM.

### START HERE

You can work up to a longer fast by extending your fasting window gradually. Here's how to begin:

**36-HOUR FAST**
Eat dinner at 7 p.m. on day one. Skip all meals on day two. Eat breakfast at 7 a.m. on day three.

**42-HOUR FAST**
Follow the pattern above, but extend the fast on day three until 1 p.m.

intake of 200 to 250 calories). Among all fasting lengths, the study found "significant reductions in weight, abdominal circumference and blood pressure" as well as improvements in blood lipids (cholesterol and triglycerides) and glucoregulation (normalizing blood sugar and insulin). Among the 404 participants who had preexisting health complaints, 84 percent reported an improvement. Perhaps most striking, researchers found that 93 percent of subjects said they felt an increase in physical and emotional well-being and an absence of hunger, and less than 1 percent had adverse effects from their extended fasting. Their conclusion was that "periodic fasting lasting from four to 21 days is safe and well-tolerated."

### The Inside Story

Beyond being safe and achievable, prolonging a fast has been shown to intensify some of the benefits of IF in general. For example, while many people doing IF report feeling mental clarity, a study of longer fasts in the *Western Journal of Medicine* found that "the subjective psychological effects of fasting may produce a sense of well-being or euphoria." That may be one reason why longer fasts seem to have such a rich spiritual and religious history.

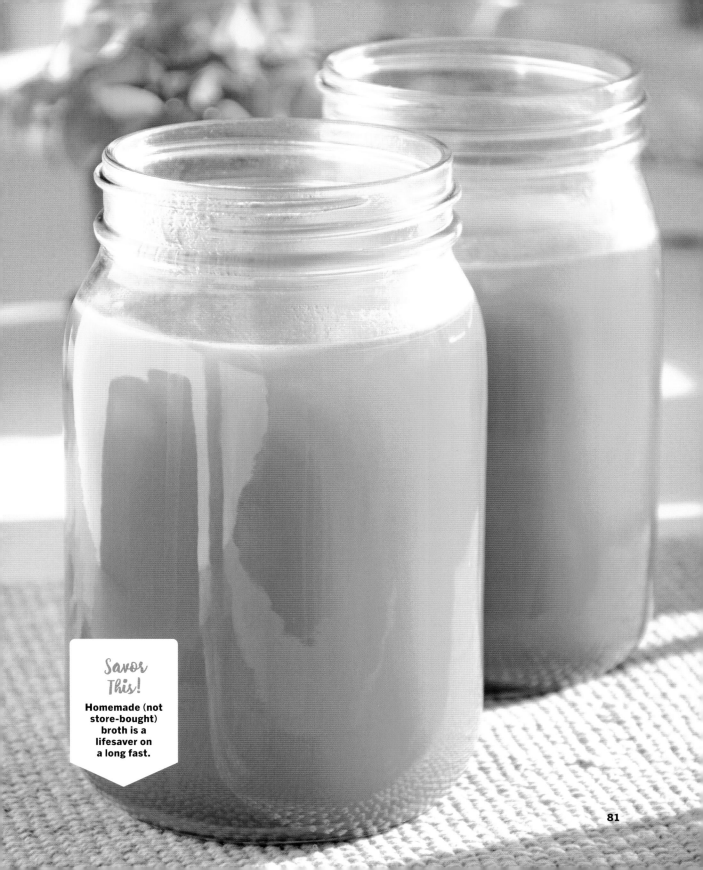

Savor This!

**Homemade (not store-bought) broth is a lifesaver on a long fast.**

81

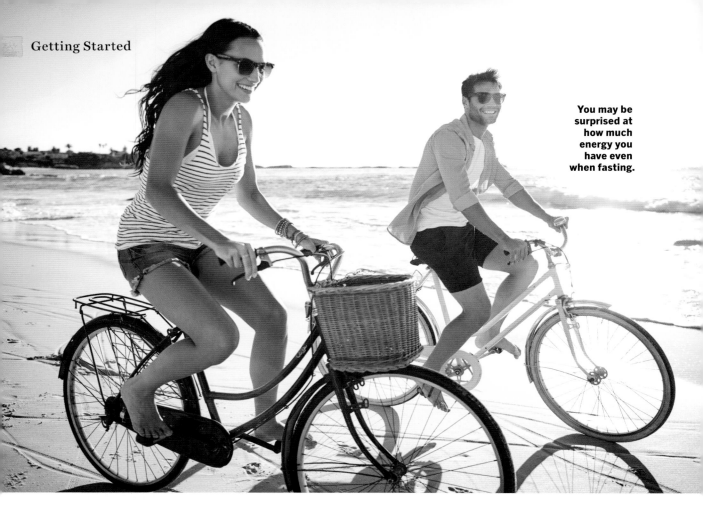

**You may be surprised at how much energy you have even when fasting.**

When it comes to increasing the body's production of human growth hormone (HGH), which all forms of IF do to some extent, extended fasts kick it into an even higher gear. One study showed that three days into a fast, HGH levels had increased by more than 300 percent, and after a week, they had increased by 1,250 percent. Other studies have found similar effects, with double or triple HGH levels after just two to three days of fasting. One trigger for this is that the presence of glucose inhibits the secretion of growth hormone; once glucose falls to almost zero, HGH really ramps up. In an evolutionary sense, this may occur because when the body senses a lack of fuel, it goes into "repair" mode to make sure that functioning can continue. So all your cells are getting a boost, with dysfunctional cells being cleared out and replaced with fresh ones.

Another intriguing benefit is that longer fasts may increase the effectiveness of cancer treatments, while reducing side effects. A study in the *Oman Medical Journal* found that normal cells that are "starved" by fasting go into a "protective mode," while cancer cells, because they are mutated, are not similarly protected against stress. The study concluded that "fasting results in overall reduction in chemotherapy side effects in cancer patients."

## The Hunger-Hormone Switch

The greatest concern most people have about extending a fast is hunger—won't it just be unbearable? A lot of evidence answers a clear no, says Ramos, who works with many clients doing extended fasts and has done several herself. In some ways, shorter fasts are more difficult than longer ones, she says, because your body doesn't have enough time to truly get into fat-burning mode. "Once you access your fat stores, you're providing your body with a lot of fuel," Ramos says. And fat as fuel is more satiating than carbs and glucose, so it's almost like a cruise-control feeding of your body internally. "Many people find that after a longer fast, when they go to eat they're just not that hungry," says Ramos.

One reason for the drop in hunger is that once you enter fat-burning mode, certain counter-regulatory hormones come into play, including ghrelin, Ramos explains. Ghrelin is a hunger-inducing hormone that cycles up and down over the day with circadian rhythms, and in reaction to eating. While in the early part of a fast, ghrelin rises and you feel hungrier; it gradually falls again—and if you don't eat, it continues to fall. "We've done trials of women fasting for a period of time and we see ghrelin go to almost nothing by day three of a fast," says Ramos.

Ghrelin may even contribute to the mental clarity that fasters cite. Studies in mice have found that when ghrelin is injected, the mice perform better on learning and memory tests and show higher numbers of neuron connections in their brains. Studies of mouse brain cells grown in a dish found that adding ghrelin switched on a gene that triggers neurogenesis, a process in which brains cells multiply.

## Extending Safely

One important element of longer fasts, however, is that they require a little more oversight. You can safely plan a fast that goes to 36 or 42 hours, but if you go beyond that, consult your physician. "On an extended fast, you should seek guidance from your health care provider, especially if you're on medications for diabetes, blood pressure or other chronic conditions," says Ramos. "Some of those might need to be adjusted during a longer fast, and it's also great just to have that support."

Then, watch for warning signs: Hunger usually peaks between one and two days and then starts subsiding, but if you feel sick, weak, faint or nauseated, stop the fast and check with your doctor. Try to stay busy and keep a normal schedule—including moderate exercise—to maintain muscles and bones. And hydrate often with water, as well as tea or coffee if you like (which may help suppress hunger and boost fat burning). It also helps to consume bone broth, which contains key trace minerals, antioxidants and a little bit of protein.

## EXTENDED FASTING
### pros and cons

**PROS**

* According to anecdotal evidence as well as studies showing a decline in levels of ghrelin (an appetite-boosting hormone), you may actually become less hungry over time on a longer fast.

* You may see results—weight loss, improvements in blood sugar and inflammatory markers—more quickly, helping to boost motivation.

* Some people report a rush of "feel-good" chemicals, similar to endorphins, after the first day.

**CONS**

* Hunger, especially on the first day, can be intermittently intense.

* Some people also have side effects like headaches or difficulty sleeping.

* It's more challenging for people who are on daily medications, because many of them should be taken with food.

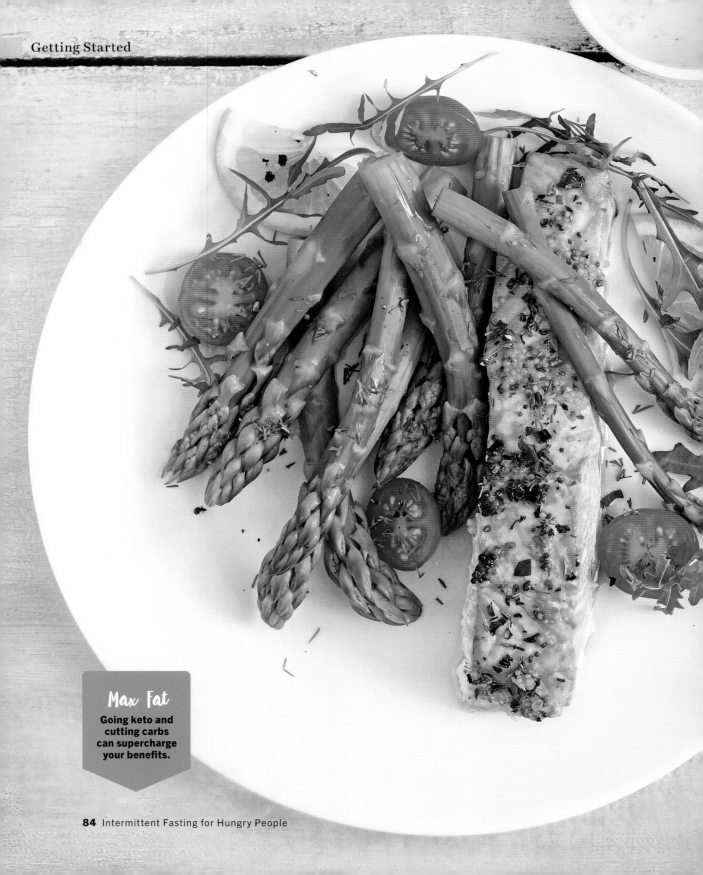

**Max Fat**

Going keto and cutting carbs can supercharge your benefits.

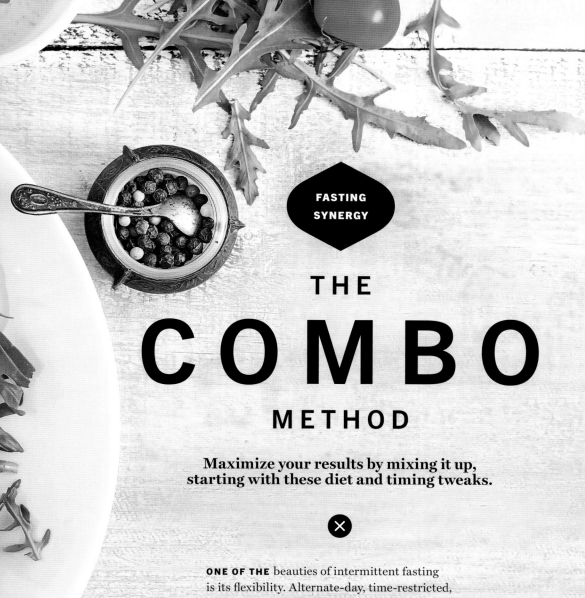

# THE
# COMBO
## METHOD

**Maximize your results by mixing it up, starting with these diet and timing tweaks.**

✕

**ONE OF THE** beauties of intermittent fasting is its flexibility. Alternate-day, time-restricted, once-a-day...they're all effective, allowing you to find the right fit for your own tastes and lifestyle. Part of that flexibility includes the question of which foods you eat during your "feasting" times. What many people like most about IF is the promise of being able to eat whatever they want when they're not fasting—although experts are quick to point out that the healthier your diet, the better your results will be.

Now, evidence is emerging that certain ways of eating, including a ketogenic diet and a carb-cycling diet, may go hand in hand with IF to

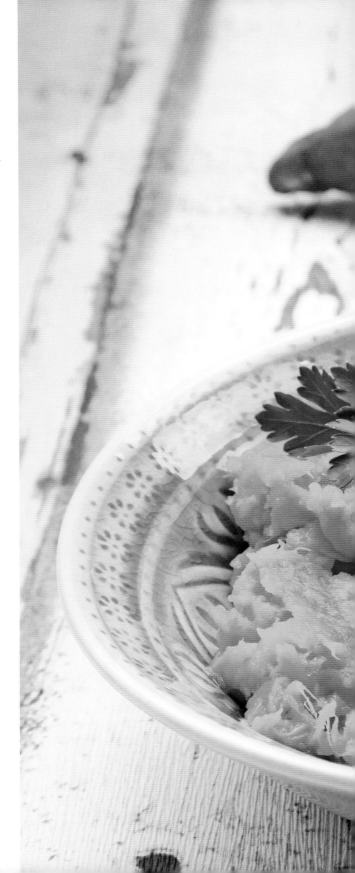

improve your weight and health even faster. While at first glance this may seem to layer on more complexity and possibly more deprivation, it turns out that keto in particular may ultimately make IF easier to carry out. Here's why.

### The Keto Advantage

Keto and IF are like cousins, or even like siblings—they both ultimately work by a similar mechanism, says Kristin Hoddy, PhD, RDN, who has extensively studied IF. "In both scenarios, your body is forced to use fat as a fuel source," Hoddy explains. "During 'fasting ketosis,' fat stores from all over your body are used as fuel. During a ketogenic diet, your body enters 'nutritional ketosis' and relies on the high fat in your diet, and the ketones you make, for fuel."

Bottom line: Both keto and IF shift your body over from using glucose for fuel to using fat for fuel. When you're fasting, you run out of stored glucose and must turn to stored fat for energy; on keto, you've lowered your carb intake so far that, again, you must access fat stores and also start creating ketones—an alternate fuel that is especially key to supplying your brain. This fuel-shifting is intimately connected to insulin, which is released when you eat (and even more so when you eat carbs), and whose purpose is in part to encourage fat storage. When insulin goes down in the absence of food (fasting) or carbs (keto), fat gets released from your body for burning.

So it's not surprising, really, that keto and IF can work well together. A century ago, when a ketogenic diet was found to help children with epilepsy, says Hoddy, "an initial fast prior to a

✕

## A HIGH-FAT DIET LIKE KETO CAN HELP KEEP HUNGER PANGS AT BAY.

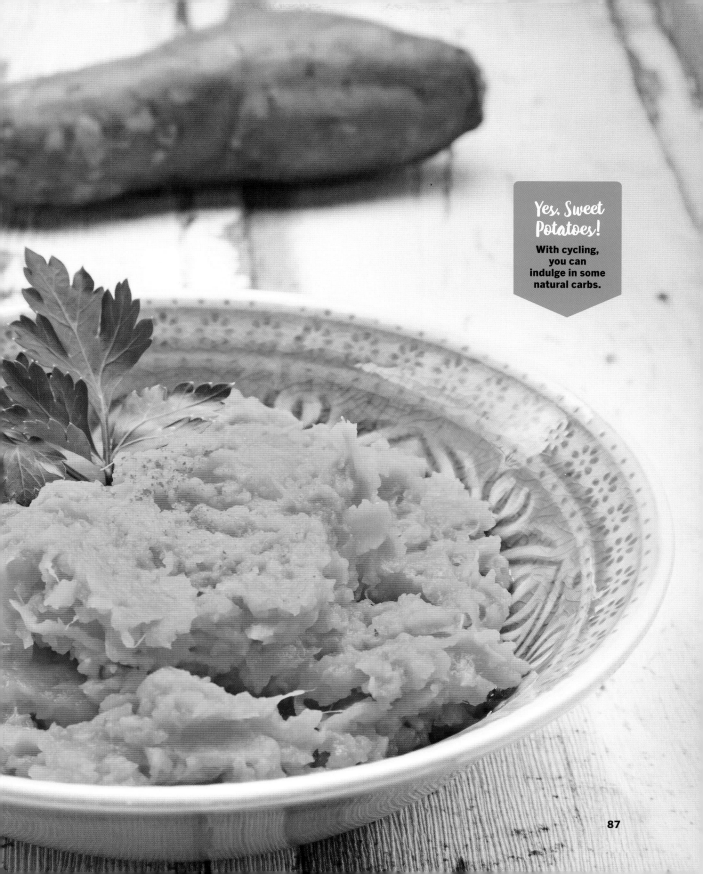

Yes, Sweet
Potatoes!

**With cycling,
you can
indulge in some
natural carbs.**

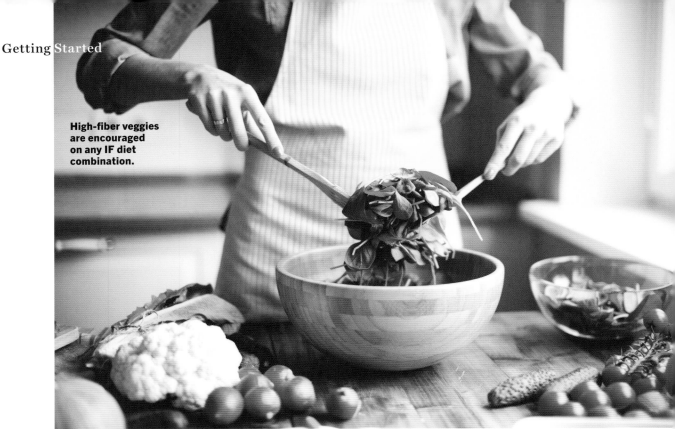

**High-fiber veggies are encouraged on any IF diet combination.**

ketogenic diet was used to kick-start ketosis in the children." And today, some people kick off an IF regimen with a so-called "fat fast," which is like keto on steroids—a period of eating almost zero carbs and lots of fat, to give a head start to the insulin drop and fat-burning that comes with IF. Think of it this way: All foods prompt some release of insulin, but carbs (especially the simple, processed kinds) cause a higher rush of insulin. So refraining from eating for periods of time, and then eating very few carbs when you do, is like a double whammy for weight loss.

## The Hunger Component

There's another compelling reason to combine keto and IF, which is that it may make fasting easier to accomplish. "I highly recommend the combination of a very low-carb diet with intermittent fasting," says Ted Naiman, MD, co-author of *The P:E Diet*. "The closer you get to a ketogenic diet—extremely low in carbohydrates,

moderate in protein and high in fat—the easier it is to go for hours and hours without eating." That's due in part to the fact that keto helps your body become "fat-adapted," Naiman explains, meaning you've built pathways to more easily access your fat stores. So rather than going hungry, your body knows where to go to get fuel.

Regarding that hunger thing: Numerous studies have shown that a keto diet is more satiating than a low-fat one, and that it can tamp down appetite. A study in *PLOS ONE* in 2018 found that a high-fat or high-protein meal had a markedly different effect on hunger-influencing hormones than a high-carb meal did. Six hours after eating lots of fat or protein, subjects had higher levels of the satiety hormones PYY and GLP-1 than the high-carb eaters did. Conversely, high-fat and high-protein meals lowered levels of the appetite-stimulating hormone ghrelin more than high-carb meals did. The result, for keto eaters, is a greater feeling of fullness and a tamed appetite.

Another study, this one a meta-analysis that evaluated a larger body of evidence, found that people following a keto diet reported feeling less hungry and had a "reduced desire to eat." The authors pointed out that this was especially remarkable considering that the subjects were on a weight-loss diet, which is notorious for inducing a serious case of the munchies. It may be that the shift in hunger hormones induced by a keto diet combines with the inherent satiating effect of fat and protein—which are digested more slowly than carbs—to keep you satisfied for longer.

## The Cycle Plan

At the core of IF is the idea of surprising your body. Rather than getting its regularly scheduled and predictable three meals plus snacks, your system has to stay on its toes to react to different feeding times. Just like when you change up your workouts to induce muscle confusion, this ultimately makes your body stronger. That's the thinking behind the idea of carb cycling. Ori Hofmekler, a former member of the Israeli Special Forces who introduced the idea of the Warrior diet almost 20 years ago, describes his system for cycling in and out of a carb-based versus a protein-and-fat-based diet in his book *The Warrior Diet*. The plan calls for one meal a day, in the afternoon or evening. Hofmekler recommends making one or two days a higher-carb day—natural ones like potatoes and whole grains, not processed carbs like muffins. Then, the next one to two days are weighted toward healthy fats and protein—such as olive oil, avocado, chicken and fish. Cycling allows you to eat a healthy variety of foods, and satisfy cravings for natural carbs, while throwing your body a curveball that keeps it tuned up and reactive.

Another form of cycling is to mix and match different kinds of fasts. For instance, you could follow a 16:8 plan in which you eat within an

## What to Eat on Keto

The basics are simple and straightforward: Tilt your diet toward high fat and moderate protein, and cut almost all carbs. That means not just the obvious ones like bread and pasta, but high-carb fruits and vegetables like bananas, potatoes and beets. Here's a quick checklist of keto do's and don'ts.

| DO EAT | DON'T EAT |
|---|---|
| Nuts | Grains (bread, rice, couscous) |
| Avocado | Pasta |
| Olives | Legumes |
| Eggs | High-carb vegetables (potatoes, carrots, parsnips, corn, beets) |
| Meat | |
| Fish | |
| Chicken | **PUT A FORK IN IT** Steer clear of the simple carbs found in plain white pasta. |
| High-fat dairy (cream, cheese, butter) | |
| Low-carb vegetables (leafy greens, cauliflower, broccoli, zucchini) | |

eight-hour window on most days, and then throw in a 24-hour fast once a week. Or you could try one day of a Warrior or one-meal-a-day (OMAD) plan. Again, the changeup keeps your body from getting into a rut, and also keeps your interest from flagging—a win-win all around.

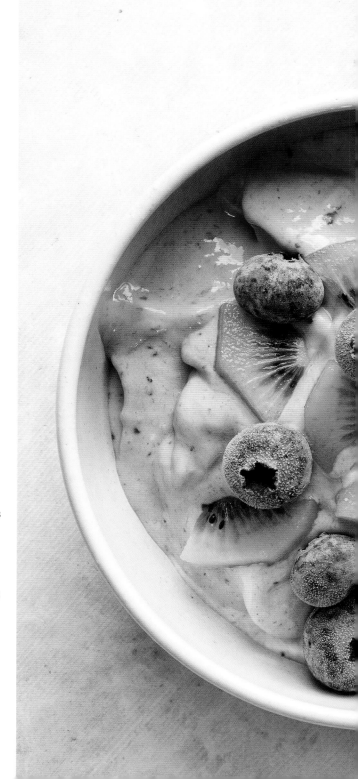

# BREAKING
# THE
# FAST

**What you eat after running
on empty—and how much you eat—
is a key part of the process.
Follow these pointers to do it
safely and enjoyably.**

**THERE'S ONE THING** that virtually every faster
agrees on: Food usually tastes amazing when you
start eating again. Kelsey, 27, says the meal she
ate at 8 p.m. on her first day of the Warrior plan
"tasted like the best dinner I'd ever had." Michael
Mosley, MD, author of *The Fast Diet* and a 5:2
faster, raves about his fast-breaking meal: "Flavors
sing and mouthfuls dance. There's nothing like
delayed gratification to make things taste good."

Historically, breaking a fast has meant
"breakfast," that meal after an overnight fast—
although if you're one of the millions of Americans
who have a late-night snack, be it popcorn or ice
cream, that fast is likely to be less than 10 or so
hours. But with IF, fasts break at many different
times. A 16:8 faster will likely have the first meal
of the day around noon or 1 p.m. Someone on
the 5:2 plan will break their fast in the morning

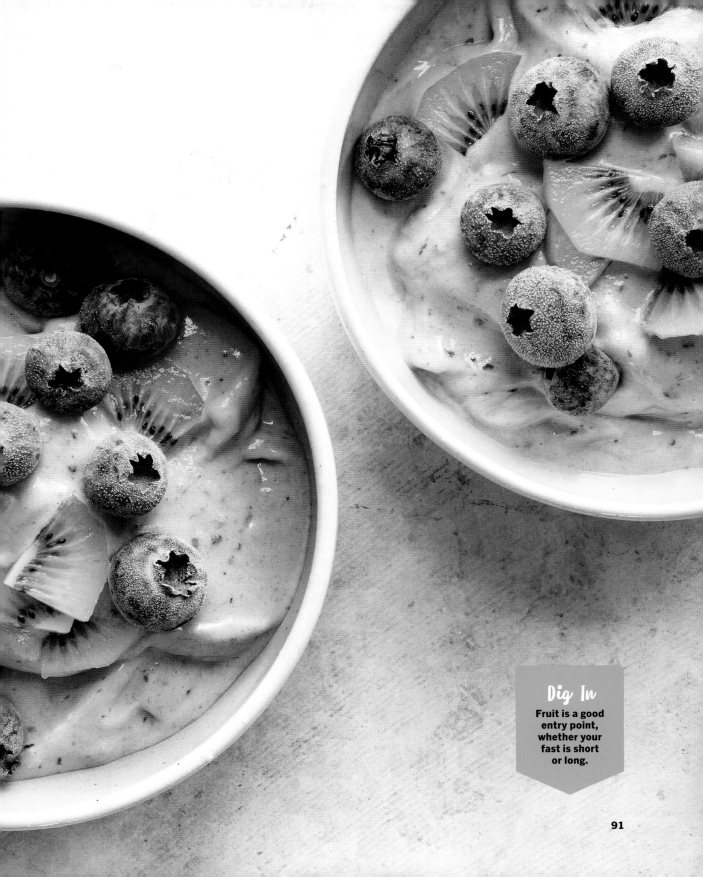

### Dig In

**Fruit is a good entry point, whether your fast is short or long.**

91

after a 500-calorie day. The Warrior faster breaks it with a full dinner. And each will have a somewhat different experience. There are some general guidelines, however, that can apply to anyone coming off a fast.

## 1 Don't Overeat

The odd thing is, most people don't. "We've run close to 700 people through various trials," says Krista Varady, PhD, a professor of nutrition at the University of Illinois at Chicago. "We thought people would overeat on their feast days to compensate. But people, for some reason, regardless of their body weight, can only eat about 10 or 15 percent more than usual. They don't really overeat, and I think that's why this works." Other studies have shown that while people ending a fast may eat somewhat more at their first meal, by the end of the day their intake has fallen. That said, you do risk stomach upset if you dive into a large meal while coming off a fast, and you risk negating the effects of fasting if you consider your eating window to be an all-out food fest. "You can't expect to trim down by skipping one meal, then making up for it at the next one," says Julian Whitaker, MD, author of *The Ultimate Guide to Intermittent Fasting*. "Gluttony will undermine any program." Listen to your satiety cues as you savor your meal.

## 2 Start Slow

This is related to point No. 1 above, because eating slowly allows you to gauge your level of fullness much more accurately. Chew your food thoroughly, advises Chelsey Amer, RD, ideally chewing each bite at least 30 times. This gives your whole system a chance to adjust to being fed again. Amer suggests having a small meal or large snack—say, a bowl of soup, or a slice of whole-wheat toast with cream cheese and smoked salmon—and then waiting an hour or two and checking your hunger level again. If you're doing 16:8, this could mean your noon meal is a couple of scrambled eggs with a piece of toast and some fruit, with a larger meal closer to dinnertime. On the Warrior plan, it translates into having an appetizer or two and letting some time go by before diving into your large dinner. And on 5:2, rather than starting with a huge breakfast on the day after a fast day, make it moderately sized: yogurt and berries, or oatmeal with bananas. Follow up with a more expansive lunch.

## 3 Eat Healthy (But Eat What You Want.)

There's no rule about what your fast-breaking meal or snack should look like. Alicia, 28, who lost more than 100 pounds on a combination of IF and a high-protein/moderate-carb diet, follows 16:8 and opens her eating window at noon with a chicken salad with French dressing. Senitha, 21, who combined keto, weight training and IF to lose 50 pounds, prefers a more breakfast-like noon meal. "I love to have an egg scramble with spinach, a side of bacon and avocado," she says. You may want to consider having more cooked foods than raw for your first meal, says Amer: Cooked vegetables are easier to digest than raw ones. And always include a protein source, adds Whitaker: "Protein minimizes insulin secretion and helps control appetite, so try to include protein-rich items with all meals and snacks." Avoid refined carbs and processed foods, as even within an IF framework these foods cause blood sugar and insulin spikes, and up your veggie intake as much as possible—they're fiber-rich, filling and loaded with nutrients.

## But What About Breakfast?

Having a morning meal makes a lot of intuitive sense: After all, you need energy from food to start the day and function at your best. If you skip it, you'll binge on bad stuff later. As the saying goes, you should eat breakfast like a king, lunch like a prince and dinner like a pauper. If you eat

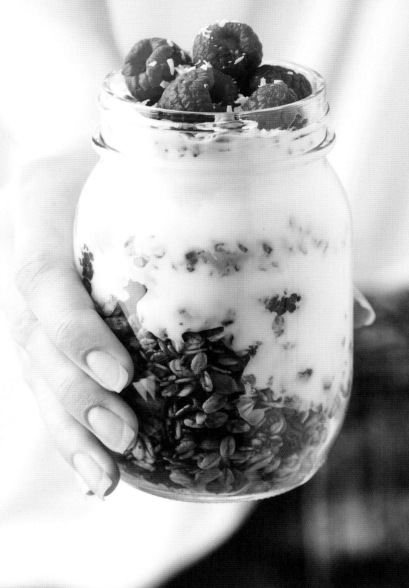

**FASTING CAN MAKE YOU APPRECIATE THE FLAVOR OF EVERY BITE YOU TAKE.**

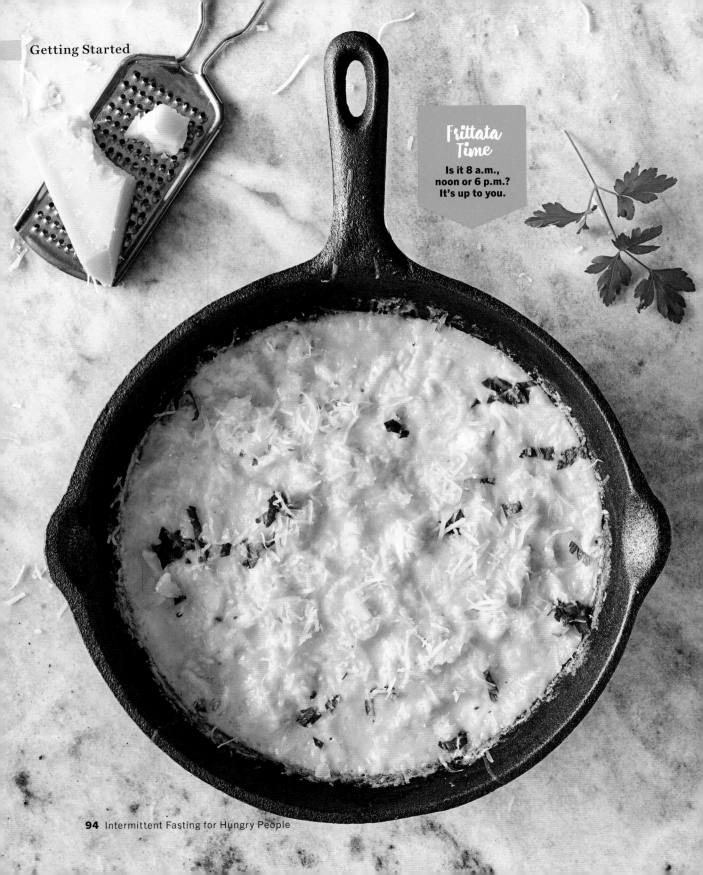

### Frittata Time

**Is it 8 a.m., noon or 6 p.m.? It's up to you.**

more later in the day, the calories will just "sit there" and turn to fat, while if you eat early, you'll burn off the calories. The problem is that all the evidence about fasting—and emerging evidence about eating first thing in the morning—turns these bromides upside down.

In fact, around a third of people in developed countries skip breakfast, points out Tim Spector, MD, professor of genetic epidemiology at King's College London. That's partly because many people simply aren't hungry for breakfast, perhaps due to the circadian rhythms of the hunger hormone, ghrelin. That hormone, which drives appetite, is lowest at 8 a.m. and peaks to its highest levels at 8 p.m. At the same time, insulin sensitivity is highest in the morning. Some have used that fact to urge breakfast-eating, on the rationale that the calories you consume in the a.m. will be used more efficiently. Here's the thing, though: "In the morning," in the case of insulin, really means "after a period of overnight fasting." If you prolong that fasting period, you'll have an even more beneficial effect on insulin sensitivity—something that has been shown in people following the 16:8 IF plan.

Comprehensive studies are finally catching up to the idea of saying no to breakfast. One meta-analysis of 13 randomized controlled trials looking at breakfast-eating and weight found that people assigned to eat breakfast had a higher overall daily calorie intake—meaning that breakfast skippers did not compensate for the "skipped" calories later in the day. It also found that those assigned to skip breakfast weighed slightly less than the breakfast eaters, flying in the face of earlier claims that to lose weight, you should be sure to eat breakfast.

It may be that many earlier studies, most of which were observational rather than clinical, had confounding factors. For instance, says Spector, "multiple observational studies have shown that obese and diabetic people skipped meals more often than thin people." But that is an association, not a cause-and-effect, and could be due to any number of factors, including guilt about overeating the night before. Similarly, observational studies have shown that breakfast-eating may be reflective of a wider healthy lifestyle; people who are more health-conscious and of higher socioeconomic status are more likely to eat breakfast because they want to make "healthy food choices." Take those same people and put them on a 16:8 fasting plan that skips breakfast, and they will likely be just as healthy—if not more so.

As far as hunger, many people find that they feel hungrier if they *do* eat breakfast, especially if it was largely carb-based (as is typical in the U.S., with choices like bagels, cereals and pastries), which triggers an insulin surge, says Whitaker. "I emphasize forgoing breakfast because many people find it's easier that way," he adds. "You've already been fasting for 10 to 12 hours, much of it while asleep, without even trying. Avoiding food for long stretches during the day requires discipline." Whitaker advises having coffee or tea to get your day started and skipping breakfast. And if you love omelets and bacon, he adds, "Do what I do—eat 'breakfast' for lunch or dinner." Lastly, if you're an early bird who feels like you can't function until noon without food, you don't have to stick to the common eating window of between noon and 8 p.m. Try eating all your meals between, say, 10 a.m. and 6 p.m.

✕

APOLOGIES TO MOMS EVERYWHERE, BUT MORNING MEALS AREN'T ESSENTIAL.

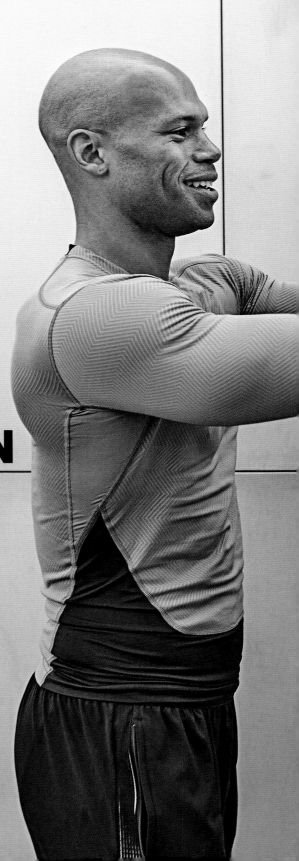

Chapter

# 3

×

# FINDING INSPIRATION

**WINNING GAME PLANS,
SUCCESS STORIES AND MORE.**

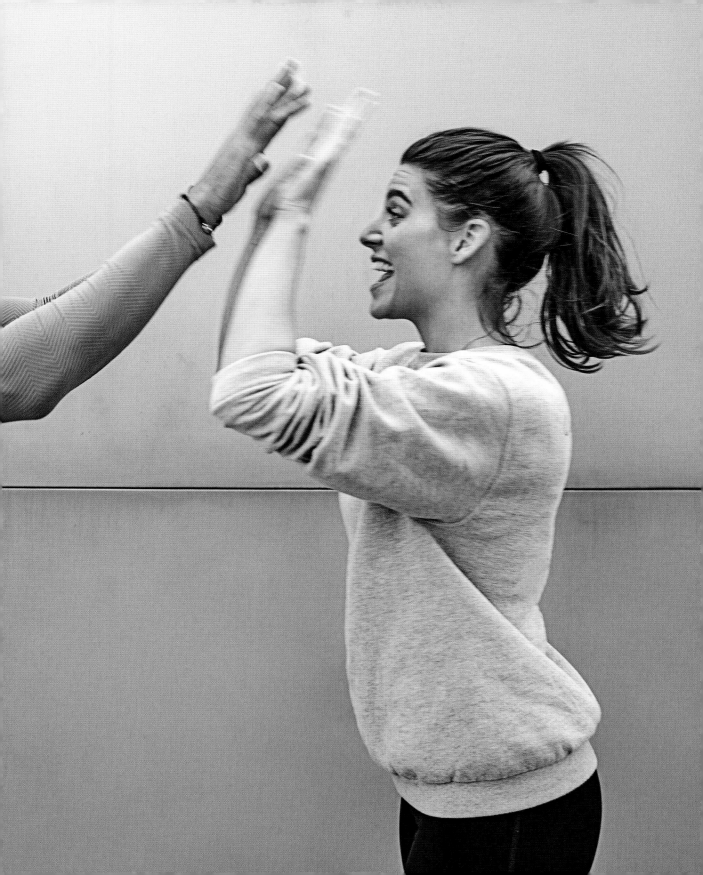

# 5 WAYS TO
# JUMP-START
## YOUR FAST

**For many people, the first few days of fasting are the most daunting—but they don't need to be, if you use these strategies.**

**THE FIRST THING** to remember about intermittent fasting is this: It's not a diet, it's a pattern of eating. It's helpful to remind yourself of this fact as you prepare to embark on an IF plan, because the very concept of a "diet" implies a short-term intervention—a period of deprivation that will land you on the lower end of the scale, at which point you can return to your old habits (a line of reasoning that helps explain why more than 90 percent of dieters regain the weight they've lost). IF is the opposite of that: It's a long-term way of life that ideally becomes second nature, woven into your schedule and familiar to your body.

With that in mind, prepping for an IF lifestyle should be done with deliberation. If you lay your foundation well, you'll have a much better chance of making IF a true new beginning, and living your life on a different—and healthier—schedule.

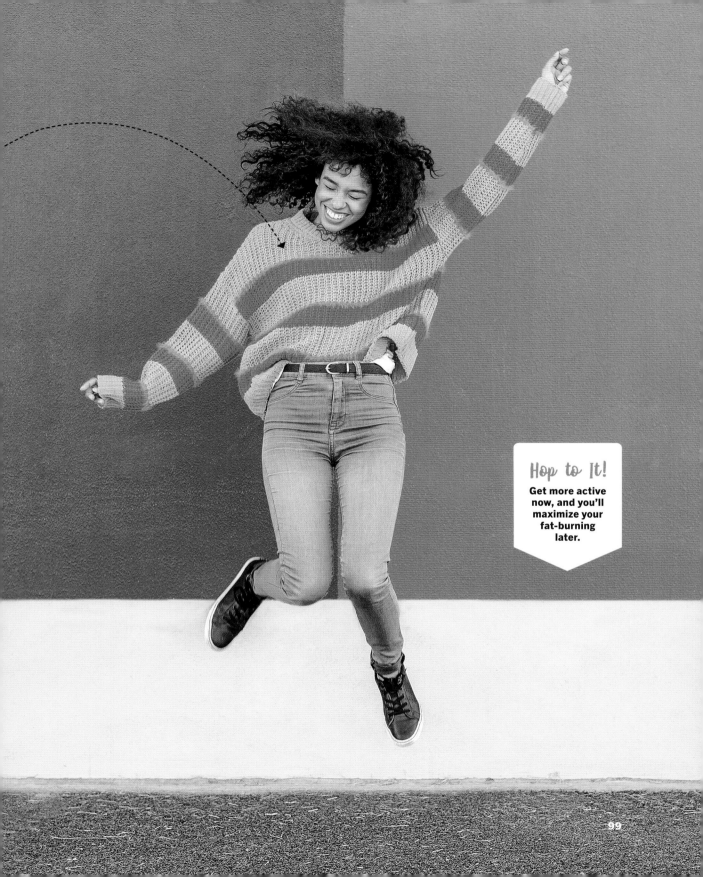

Hop to It!
Get more active now, and you'll maximize your fat-burning later.

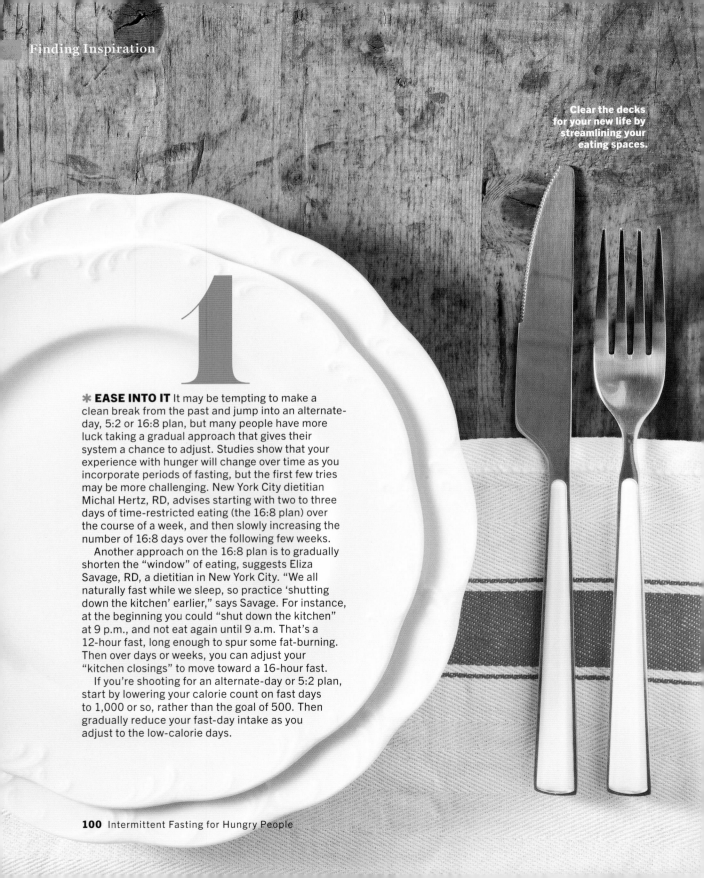

Clear the decks for your new life by streamlining your eating spaces.

# 1

✳ **EASE INTO IT** It may be tempting to make a clean break from the past and jump into an alternate-day, 5:2 or 16:8 plan, but many people have more luck taking a gradual approach that gives their system a chance to adjust. Studies show that your experience with hunger will change over time as you incorporate periods of fasting, but the first few tries may be more challenging. New York City dietitian Michal Hertz, RD, advises starting with two to three days of time-restricted eating (the 16:8 plan) over the course of a week, and then slowly increasing the number of 16:8 days over the following few weeks.

Another approach on the 16:8 plan is to gradually shorten the "window" of eating, suggests Eliza Savage, RD, a dietitian in New York City. "We all naturally fast while we sleep, so practice 'shutting down the kitchen' earlier," says Savage. For instance, at the beginning you could "shut down the kitchen" at 9 p.m., and not eat again until 9 a.m. That's a 12-hour fast, long enough to spur some fat-burning. Then over days or weeks, you can adjust your "kitchen closings" to move toward a 16-hour fast.

If you're shooting for an alternate-day or 5:2 plan, start by lowering your calorie count on fast days to 1,000 or so, rather than the goal of 500. Then gradually reduce your fast-day intake as you adjust to the low-calorie days.

✕

## LOW-GLYCEMIC FOODS LIKE VEGGIES AND WHOLE GRAINS PROVIDE A METABOLIC ADVANTAGE WHEN CUTTING CALORIES.

**✳ CHECK IN WITH YOUR DOC** One reason for having a checkup is that it gives you a starting point to gauge your progress. You'll get your weight, blood pressure and blood panel measured, to see where you stand on cholesterol and blood sugar—all stats that will likely improve once you start IF. But a doctor's visit will also alert you to any potential issues, says Tro Kalayjian, MD, who runs Dr. Tro's Medical Weight Loss program in Tappan, New York. "You may have medical conditions that need monitoring," he cautions. "Or be on medications that need to be adjusted. It's important to have an understanding of your medical history before starting a fasting program."

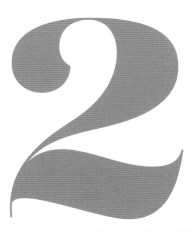

**✳ START CUTTING CARBS BEFOREHAND**
Fasting experts agree that going straight from a high-carb, sweet- and starch-filled diet to an IF regimen is especially challenging. That's because a high-carb diet (including the typical American diet) has conditioned your body for frequent cycles of insulin release and blood sugar ups and downs. So when you switch to IF and your insulin naturally falls, it can feel like a bigger crash. Also, because carbs are broken down so quickly in the body, you tend to feel hungry more often. In contrast, a higher-fat diet is more satiating, and can also lower your insulin pre-fast, giving you a jump-start.

Consider kicking your toast, cereal and pasta habit to the curb, and replacing those simple carbs with eggs, cheese, meat and nonstarchy vegetables, starting in the weeks or month before trying your first fast. You'll be in much better nutritional standing to make IF work for you.

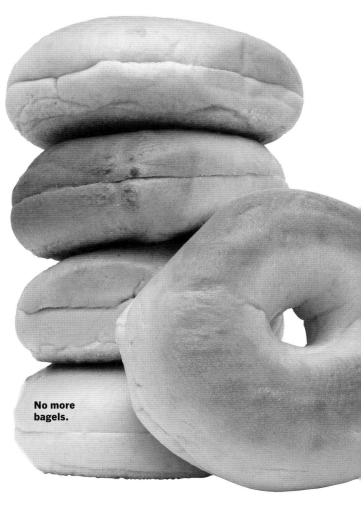

No more bagels.

## 4

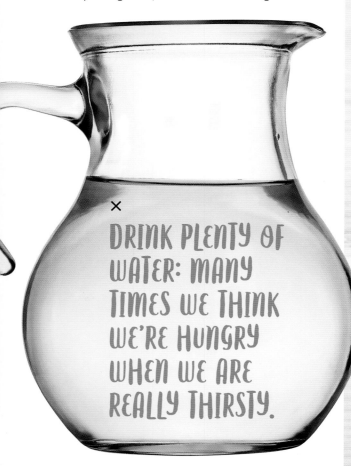

✳ **CLEAN HOUSE** You know how tough it is to *not* eat the Oreo when it's staring you in the face! Go through your fridge and cupboards and toss your trigger foods. We eat for many reasons besides hunger, points out Michael Mosley, MD, author of *The Fast Diet*. "We eat when we're bored, when we're thirsty, when we're around food, when we're with company or simply when the clock tells us it's time for food." Make those reflexive hunger pangs harder to indulge by removing obvious temptations from your cupboards. Instead, stock up on herbal teas, sparkling water, flavored coffee and organic broth.

×

## DRINK PLENTY OF WATER: MANY TIMES WE THINK WE'RE HUNGRY WHEN WE ARE REALLY THIRSTY.

## 5

✳ **TRY A FAT FAST FIRST** A so-called fat fast is like Rule No. 2 in overdrive. "The idea is to eat lots of fatty foods until satiated for a few days before you start fasting," explains Megan Ramos, co-founder of the Intensive Dietary Management Program. "This helps your body reach fat-burning mode faster and without as much hunger." A fat fast is especially helpful when coming off a period of eating a mostly high-carb diet, when you're already full of cravings, or during times of stress when trying IF seems practically impossible.

The rules of a fat fast are simple, says Ramos: Eat when hungry and until full, as often as necessary. Avoid dairy and nuts; focus on eggs, bacon, salmon, sardines and fat sources like olive oil, coconut oil, butter, mayo, avocados and olives. Limiting food choices is one reason this plan is helpful, Ramos says—and you'll only be eating this way for a few days. "There are two reasons the fat fast works," she explains. "It's an extreme version of a ketogenic diet, and the monotony of the limited foods suppresses your appetite. And fat is extremely satiating." You'll also have removed insulin-spiking carbs and laid the foundation for fat-burning.

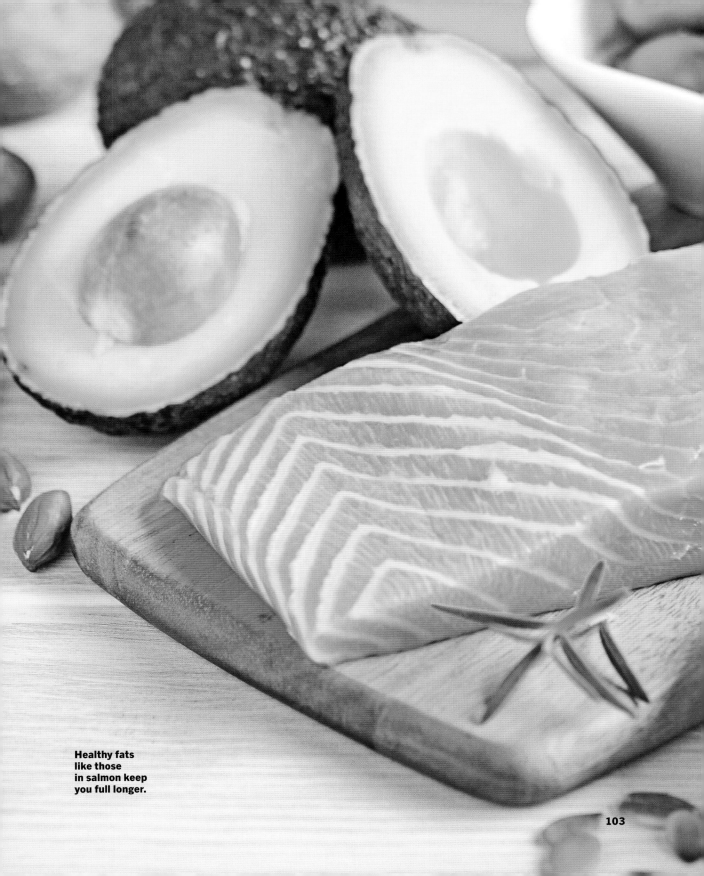

Healthy fats
like those
in salmon keep
you full longer.

# FIRST-RATE
# FARE

**Fasting puts the focus on what you *do* eat. So fill your tank— and boost your energy—with these powerhouse foods.**

**INTERMITTENT FASTING MAY** be all about avoiding food, but the inverse is also true: IF makes your food choices even more important. When you're grazing often, it can be easier to add in some antioxidants here and fiber sources there. Clustering your eating occasions into smaller windows means your noshes take on greater significance, since you only have so many hours in which to ensure a well-rounded diet. Your choices are also key because certain foods bump up your results by supplying satiating fats and fiber, feeding your microbiome (the microbes that live inside the body) and helping reduce inflammation. Start by putting these superfoods on your feast-time menu.

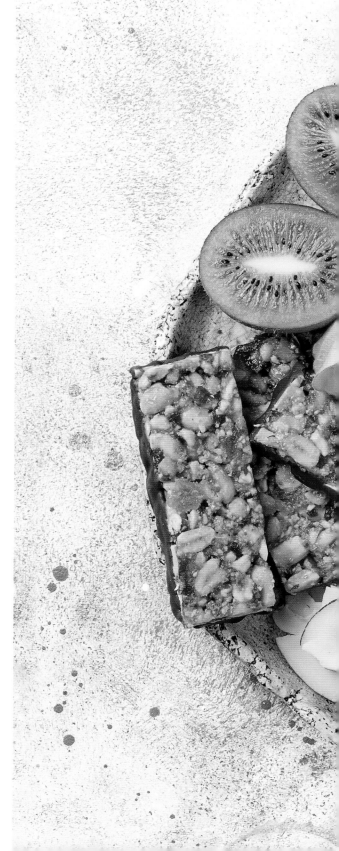

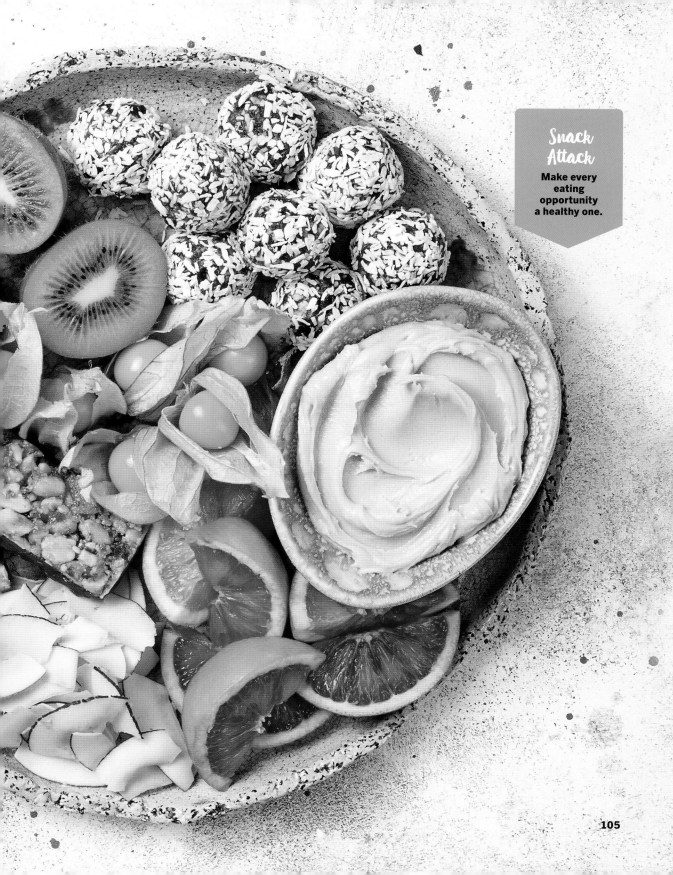

Snack
Attack

**Make every
eating
opportunity
a healthy one.**

# ARTiCHOKE

A single artichoke has a whopping 7 grams of fiber, which is twice as much as you'd get from a cup of cooked cauliflower. "Artichokes contain prebiotic fibers that are essential to your gut health," says Naomi Whittel, author of *High Fiber Keto*. "Fiber literally 'feeds' your gut bacteria, helping to keep your microbiome in balance and the good bacteria in charge. That's critical to your overall health, and especially your metabolic health." Fasting gives your digestive system a rest from its work, and when you later add in prebiotic-rich foods like artichokes, you provide your microbiome with a fresh start.

## Choke Up

Artichoke hearts are the tender baby artichokes that are picked before the prickly interior develops.

# NUT BUTTERS

Peanut butter, almond butter, cashew butter and others have a nearly ideal balance between carbs, protein and fats. And those fats are the healthy kind—mostly monounsaturated, along with omega-3 and omega-6 fatty acids. Not only are they satiating, but they may help account for nuts' health benefits. Numerous studies have shown that people who eat nuts live longer than those who don't, perhaps because nuts appear to help prevent a number of chronic diseases, especially metabolic syndrome and cardiovascular disease. Time to whip up a peanut butter sandwich!

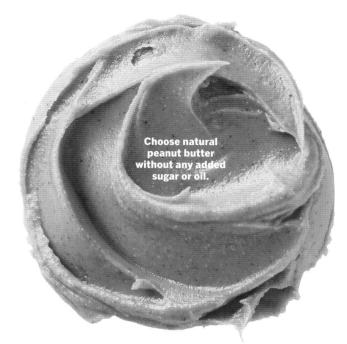

**Choose natural peanut butter without any added sugar or oil.**

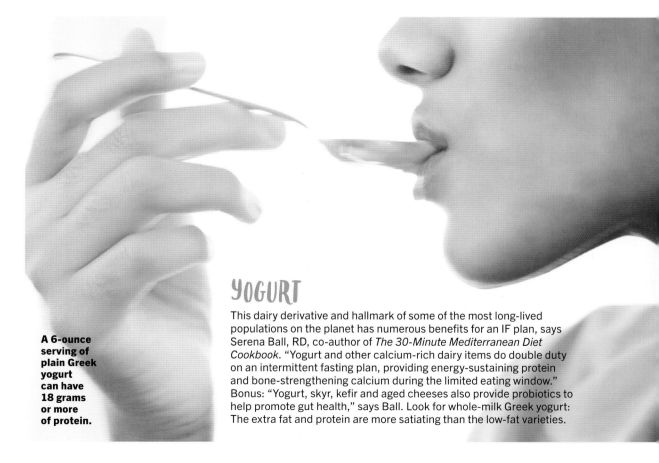

# YOGURT

This dairy derivative and hallmark of some of the most long-lived populations on the planet has numerous benefits for an IF plan, says Serena Ball, RD, co-author of *The 30-Minute Mediterranean Diet Cookbook*. "Yogurt and other calcium-rich dairy items do double duty on an intermittent fasting plan, providing energy-sustaining protein and bone-strengthening calcium during the limited eating window." Bonus: "Yogurt, skyr, kefir and aged cheeses also provide probiotics to help promote gut health," says Ball. Look for whole-milk Greek yogurt: The extra fat and protein are more satiating than the low-fat varieties.

**A 6-ounce serving of plain Greek yogurt can have 18 grams or more of protein.**

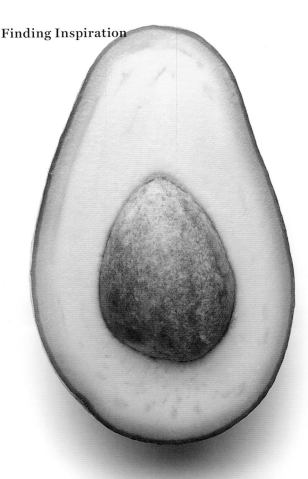

## AVOCADO

This fat- and fiber-rich fruit is a fasting star for all kinds of reasons. Not only do the 10 grams of fiber help keep you satiated, but avocados are one of the highest-fat plants in creation. An average Haas avocado has about 20 grams of fat, meaning that 77 percent of its calories are from fats—and the vast majority of those are healthy monounsaturated fatty acids that are the major component of olive oil. The high fat content not only makes you feel fuller longer, but these fatty acids are also associated with reduced inflammation and cardiovascular benefits, in part because they help raise HDL (good) cholesterol and lower LDL (bad) cholesterol. Add in sky-high potassium (more than in a banana), antioxidants, B vitamins and studies linking avocado consumption to weight loss, and you may want to whip up some avocado toast to break your fast.

✕

## KEEP AVOCADO LEFTOVERS FROM TURNING BROWN WITH A LITTLE LEMON JUICE.

## Super Snacks
### When it's time to nosh, try one of these energizing bites.

**BERRIES**
All varieties—raspberries, blueberries, strawberries and blackberries—are sky-high in antioxidants, anti-inflammatories and fiber. In addition, studies suggest that berries help increase insulin sensitivity and reduce blood sugar.

**PRUNES**
High-fiber prunes are great for digestion (and for easing constipation, a common side effect of IF), but they have other surprising benefits: They're rich in potassium, iron and boron, which strengthens bones and may help prevent osteoporosis. In addition, their low ranking on the glycemic index help keep you satisfied.

**NUTS AND SEEDS**
These little bites are loaded with satiating healthy fats and antioxidants (one study found that walnuts have a greater capacity to fight free radicals than fish does). Numerous studies have also shown that they may promote weight loss, despite being high in calories. And many varieties are super high in fiber—chia seeds have 10 grams per ounce!

**HARD-BOILED EGG**
Eggs are one of nature's near-perfect foods, packed with protein, essential fatty acids and B vitamins. To get the most benefits, shop for eggs that come from free range, organic or barn-raised chickens.

# cHOCOLaTE

As long as it's dark—at least 70 percent cacao or above—chocolate is your healthiest treat on IF. It's packed with minerals, including iron, magnesium, manganese, potassium and zinc; its fatty acid profile is excellent; and it's so rich in antioxidants that a study in the *Chemistry Central Journal* called cacao seeds a "super fruit." The study found that cacao beat out other food stars like pomegranate, blueberries, cranberries and açai for levels of health-boosting plant chemicals like polyphenol and flavonol. So when you're craving a little sweet bite after a meal or as a snack, reach for a square of the good stuff.

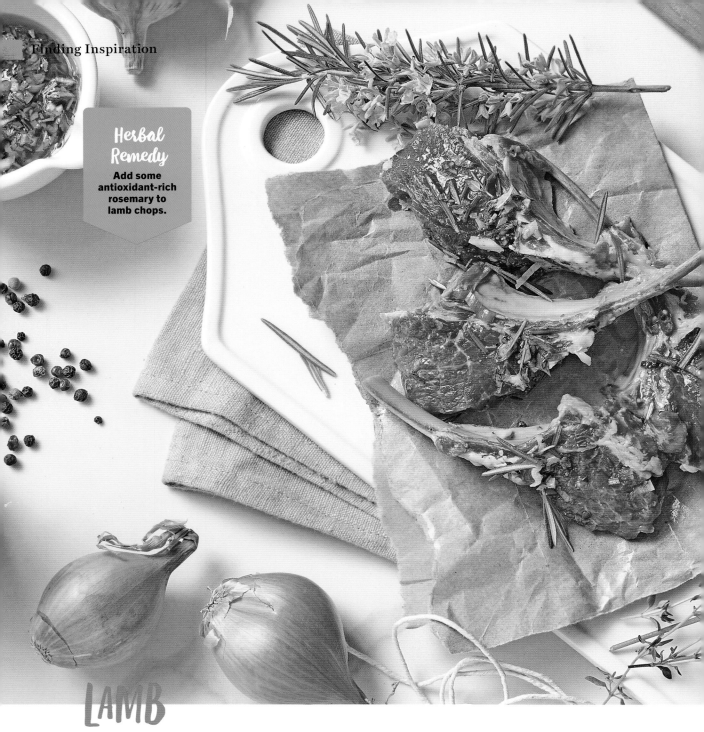

**Herbal Remedy**

**Add some antioxidant-rich rosemary to lamb chops.**

# LAMB

When it comes to meats, lamb has a special bonus, says Ball. "All lamb is grass-fed, so it's a source of beneficial CLAs, which are conjugated linoleic acids." A study in the *Journal of Dairy Science* found that CLA content is 300 to 500 percent higher in meat sources that have been grass-fed as opposed to those that were grain-fed, including beef. In mouse studies, CLAs were found to help reduce food intake, increase fat burning, stimulate fat breakdown and inhibit fat production. In addition, studies in humans have found

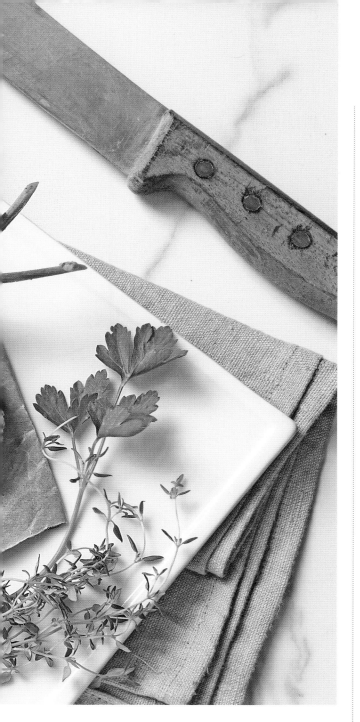

## LEAFY GREENS

Spinach, collards and other greens are packed with vitamins and antioxidants while also being very low-calorie—so portions can be unlimited. And they have another benefit that's key to IF, says Whittel: They're extra hydrating. You obtain a lot of water through foods, so fasting can leave you dehydrated. When you break your fast, pump up your $H_2O$ consumption with a form of water in foods called "gel" or "structured" water. "This has an extra hydrogen and oxygen atom, so instead of $H_2O$, it's $H_3O_2$," Whittel says, "and it's easier for your body to absorb and retain." Gel water helps hydrate your cells, fascia (connective tissue) and muscles.

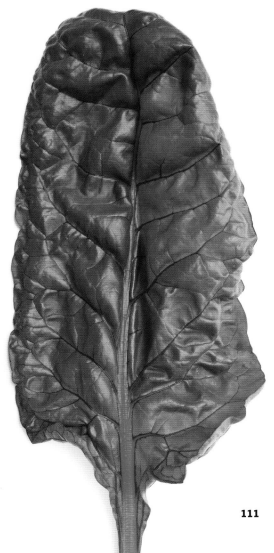

that people who take in high levels of CLA from foods are at a lower risk of various diseases, including Type 2 diabetes and cancer. Not only will high-CLA foods boost your weight loss and overall health, but grass-fed meats are full of energy-sustaining protein and iron.

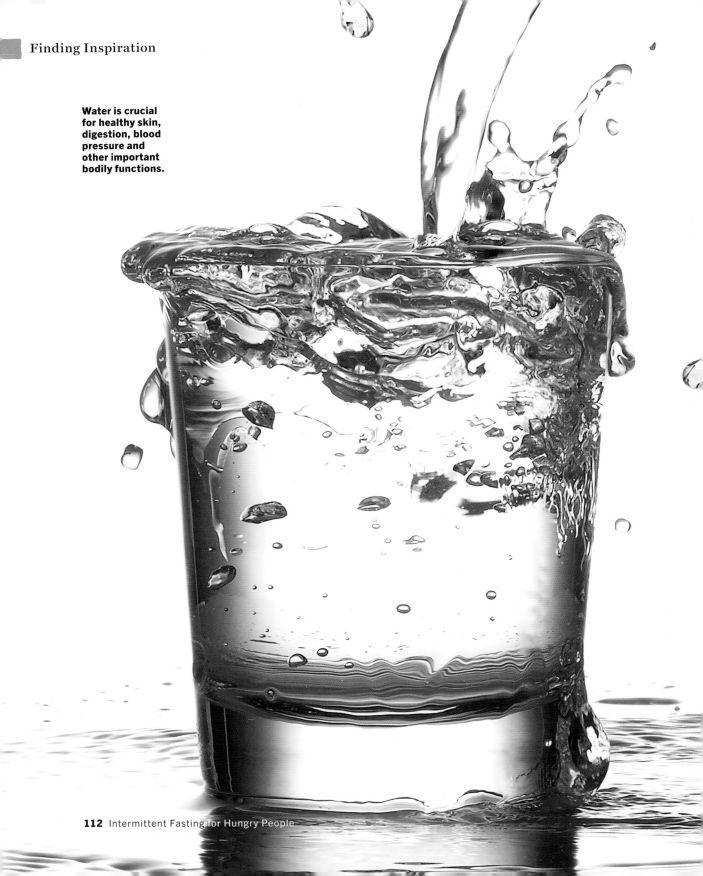

**Water is crucial for healthy skin, digestion, blood pressure and other important bodily functions.**

# LIQUID
## ASSETS

**(Almost) all things wet and wonderful are about to become your new best friends—because staying hydrated is Rule No. 1 for healthy fasting.**

**IT'S IMPOSSIBLE TO** overstate the importance of liquids in the fasting equation. First and most obvious, there's the fact that they can play an outsize role in controlling hunger, enabling you to put something in your stomach even during a fasting period. But more crucially, you get a good amount of your daily water intake from foods, explains New York City–based Keri Gans, RDN. So if you're not eating much over a period of 16 hours or on an alternate-day fasting pattern,

your body's fluids can fall far below their normal level. In addition, many side effects of fasting are connected to dehydration.

However, there's clearly a big difference between some drinks (like wine or other alcohol, or a calorie-loaded venti mocha) and fluids like herbal tea or plain old water. And there's a world of ways to make your fluid intake one of the highlights of your fast. Here's how to drink to your health.

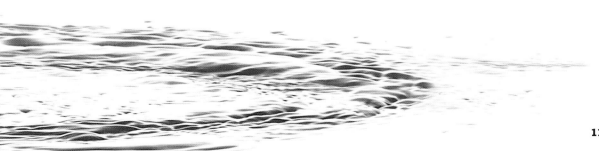

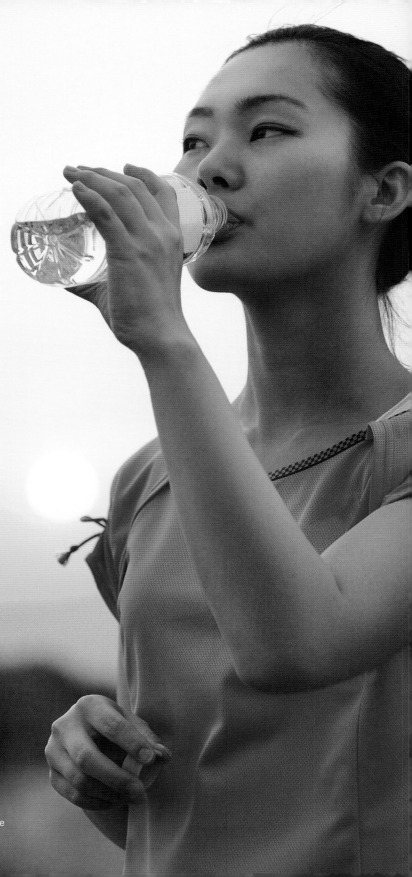

# WATER

This is always a key choice. A study in *Frontiers in Nutrition* found that, even for people who aren't fasting, increased water intake is associated with weight loss through two mechanisms: a decrease in eating and an increase in fat-burning. Mineral water may provide an extra boost, helping to mitigate any mineral imbalance—which can prompt side effects like weakness, headaches or nausea—during fasting. Aim to drink 2 liters of water and other fluids every day on IF, advises Jason Fung, MD, author of *The Obesity Code: Unlocking the Secrets of Weight Loss*. But water can be boring. A few ideas for dressing it up:

* Squeeze in some fresh lemon or lime juice.
* Fill a water pitcher and add berries or slices of cucumber, lemon or lime.
* Make herb ice cubes: Using mint, basil, rosemary or sage, put a leaf or sprig in each ice cube mold, fill about one-third of the way with water and freeze for 45 minutes (the herbs will rise to the top). Then fill the rest of the way and return to freezer.
* Go for sparkling water! The bubbles will help you feel fuller.

## WATER STAVES OFF SIDE EFFECTS WHILE BOOSTING FAT-BURNING.

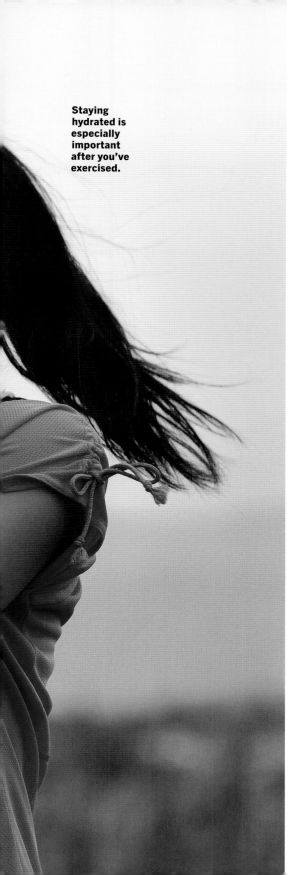

**Staying hydrated is especially important after you've exercised.**

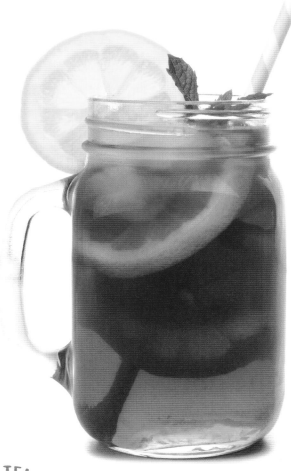

## TEA

Unsweetened tea brings many special health benefits to the table, including flavonoids: powerful antioxidants that can lower blood pressure and LDL cholesterol, and reduce the risk of cardiovascular disease. Numerous studies have shown that flavonoid-rich foods, including tea, contribute to lower total mortality. And a comprehensive study published in the journal *Nutrients* in 2019 found that tea drinkers tend to have healthier, more nutrient-rich diets and lower body mass indexes. Herbal teas (which aren't technically teas, since they're made not from tea leaves but from infusions of herbs) have their own benefits—they contain antioxidants, are anti-inflammatory, and help boost the immune and digestive systems. Chamomile is relaxing; both peppermint and ginger aid the gut and digestion; rose hip is great for the skin; echinacea helps fight a cold; and the list goes on.

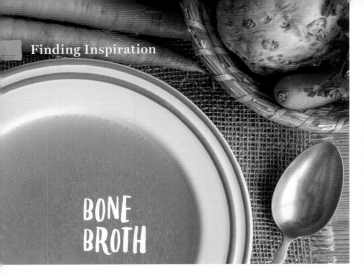

# BONE BROTH

A fasting star, bone broth contains key trace minerals, such as potassium and magnesium, which are especially beneficial during fasting, says Fung. It also contains gelatin and small amounts of protein, which help diminish hunger pangs, as well as antioxidants. Added salt is important as well, since sodium deficiency can lead to dehydration during fasting. Homemade is best, so try this simple recipe:

## HOMEMADE BONE BROTH

In a large stockpot, add:
* Bones (poultry, pork, fish, beef or lamb)
* Vegetables (chopped onion, carrots and celery)
* Sea salt
* Fresh or dried herbs or spices, if desired

Add several quarts of water, and bring to a boil; reduce heat to low. Simmer for at least four hours for fish, and several hours longer for meat or poultry. Strain out bones, veggies and fat. Store in the refrigerator for up to five days, or freeze in small containers or ice cube trays for three to four months.

## Watch Out for These
Not all drinks are equally fasting-friendly. Be careful with these:

### ALCOHOL
Avoid all alcohol during fasting periods, even on your "low-calorie" day if you're doing the 5:2 plan. Not only is alcohol just empty calories, but it hits your system hard on an empty stomach. Alcohol is permitted during the eating window—with dinner on OMAD/Warrior or 16:8, or your regular-eating days on alternate-day/5:2—but for the same empty-calorie reasons, go moderate. Avoid sugary mixers like tonic or Collins mix, and favor spirits (vodka, gin, whiskey) over carb-heavy beer and wine.

### ARTIFICIALLY SWEETENED DRINKS
Evidence has been mounting for years that artificial sweeteners like saccharin or sucralose may actually have counterproductive effects on dieters. Studies have shown that sweeteners, even without any calories, can increase insulin levels, possibly due to the sweet taste (a study with rats who were altered to remove their ability to taste found that the artificial sweeteners did not raise their insulin). That insulin spike in turn prompts cravings for actual sugar.

# COFFEE

Java is a favorite of fasters. It's full of health benefits: Many studies suggest a lowered risk of diabetes, cancer, Alzheimer's and depression, and coffee is considered the biggest source of antioxidants in the Western diet. It improves athletic performance, gives you a burst of energy—key when you feel you're flagging during a fasting period—suppresses appetite and breaks down body fat, making free fatty acids available as fuel (i.e., it bumps up your fat-burning). Like tea, you should take it unsweetened, though many fasting experts feel you won't break your fast if you add a teaspoon or two of pure fat like coconut or MCT oil (which has been shown to increase levels of satiety hormones like peptide YY and leptin). The small amount of oil may help you stave off hunger and won't stimulate an insulin response.

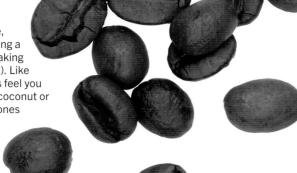

# Nature's No. 1 Sports Drink

Coconut water, made from the clear liquid inside green coconuts, is 95 percent water—but the real magic is contained in the other 5 percent. Coconut water has been consumed for centuries for its health benefits, and there are few better liquids for rehydrating post-workout. A few of its best properties compared to standard sports drinks:

**1** Unlikely to cause nausea or upset stomach

**2** Only 45 calories per cup

**3** Less sugar and carbs than most juices

**4** Has 10 times the potassium of sports drinks

**5** More calcium and magnesium (which support muscles and prevent cramps) than sports drinks

**6** Contains amino acids like alanine, arginine and cysteine, which repair tissues

**7** Contains antioxidants to neutralize oxidative stress and free radicals created by exercise

**8** Contains cytokinins, compounds believed to have anti-aging and cancer-fighting properties

**9** No dyes, synthetic ingredients or added sugars

PREMIUM Fuel

# THE
# EXERCISE
## ADVANTAGE

**Working out plus intermittent fasting
make for a powerful duo. Here's how to (safely)
get the biggest bang for your gym bucks.**

**AT FIRST GLANCE,** going for a run or lifting weights while fasting sounds counterintuitive. What about all that advice to fuel your workouts with a smoothie or a hit of protein, so you can power through at full strength? Conventional wisdom holds that you won't have a good workout on an empty stomach.

But more and more research is showing the opposite: The benefits of exercise may in fact be boosted by being in a fasting state. The most recent evidence comes from a study in the *Journal of Clinical Endocrinology and Metabolism* that compared two groups of sedentary subjects. One group consumed a protein shake two hours before a cycling session, while the other drank a placebo drink with no calories. After six weeks, the empty-stomach cyclists had burned twice as much fat as the shake-drinkers—even though both groups torched the same number of overall calories.

Not only that, but the fasting exercisers had improved insulin sensitivity and higher levels of a protein that helps muscles both respond to insulin and use blood sugar, both factors that can reduce risk of weight gain and diabetes. Even better, they didn't rate their workouts as any more draining or difficult than the shake-drinkers did.

That's good—but what happens after that fasting workout? Do a compensatory pig-out lunch and dinner follow? Logic would say yes, and research has shown that people do tend to unknowingly consume more food on days that they exercise (which may be one reason why exercise alone is rarely an effective weight-loss strategy). But working out with your tank on empty may—again, counterintuitively—short-circuit that overeating.

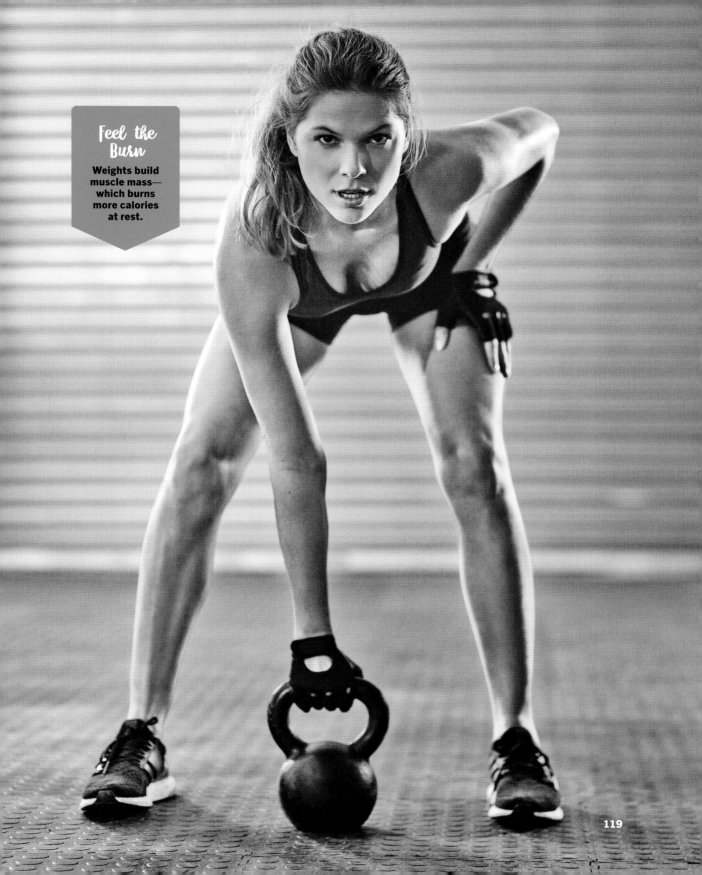

**Feel the Burn**

Weights build muscle mass—which burns more calories at rest.

# THE BEST PROGRAM IS A COMBO OF AEROBIC WORKOUTS AND STRENGTH TRAINING.

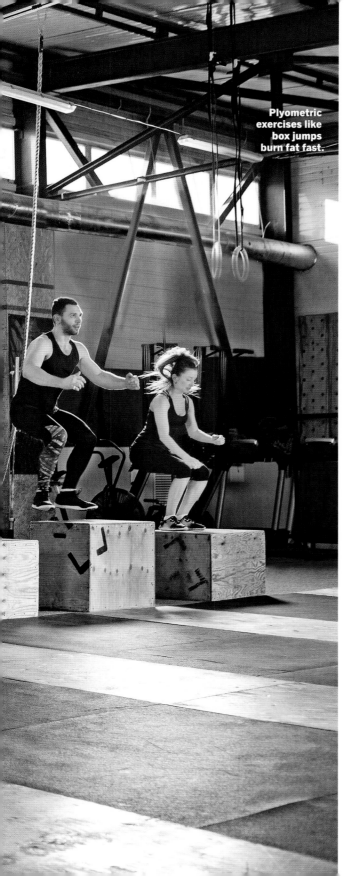

Plyometric exercises like box jumps burn fat fast.

A 2019 study in the *Journal of Nutrition* compared a group of subjects under different circumstances: First they worked out after a large oatmeal breakfast, then on another day they did the same workout in a fasting state. At lunch after the well-fed workout, the subjects' bodies balanced their energy needs precisely, burning and consuming the same number of calories over the course of a day. But after a fasting workout, while the subjects were ravenous at lunch, eating substantially more calories, their eating later trailed off. By day's end, they'd eaten 400 fewer calories than they burned—a deficit that over time could lead to weight loss.

## A Burning Question

The solution to these mysteries may lie in the kind of fuel your body burns, according to Julian Whitaker, MD, founder of the Whitaker Wellness Institute and author of *The Ultimate Guide to Intermittent Fasting*. Your body has a favorite fuel—glucose from foods—which is stored as glycogen for quick energy. This is the basis for the infamous sugar high: Glucose is burned immediately. Your body only burns fats, or ketones (an alternate energy source created by the liver), when the carb fuel runs out.

When you fast overnight, your stores of glycogen go down to fuel bodily functions, and by morning they're running low. If you don't eat something, eventually your body is forced to turn to the more labor-intensive source of energy: body fat. Picture what happens when you then start working out, says Whitaker: "You blow through your remaining glycogen and go straight into burning fat." By exercising in a fasted state, you pump up the benefits of IF (accessing fat stores after fasting 12 hours or more) and burn even more body fat, Whitaker explains. But if you snack before a workout, your body goes right to that easily accessed glucose fuel and leaves your fat cells alone. Who wouldn't want to burn off body fat rather than a protein bar?

## Kick It Up a Notch

**Want to see faster results? Once you've become fat-adapted (after at least two weeks of IF), try a high-intensity interval training (HIIT) workout. It's fast—20 minutes tops—and studies have found it improves aerobic capacity more quickly than endurance training. It has also been shown to be more effective at preserving muscle mass while reducing subcutaneous and abdominal body fat. Here, the basics of how it works.**

**1**

Choose your favorite aerobic workout (i.e. running, cycling, elliptical).

**2**

Warm up for a few minutes at a slow to moderate pace, then do 60 seconds of all-out effort—a sprint where you approach the limits of your aerobic capacity—followed by 60 seconds of recovery at a slowed pace.

**3**

Repeat for a total of 20 minutes.

**4**

Once you're adept at HIIT, you can vary the timing of the effort and recovery. Try shortening the recovery period until you're doing, say, one minute of high intensity and only 30 seconds of recovery.

**5**

Start out doing HIIT only once a week, then work up to doing HIIT every other day.

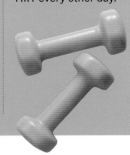

s far as why the empty-tank exercisers ate less as the day went on (after their big lunch), researchers hypothesize that our brains are tuned to pay particular attention to any reductions in our glucose levels and to urge us to replenish them. So the hungry exercisers ate a bigger lunch than usual. But that urgent "hurry up and eat" impulse may be transient, and once sated it quiets down, rather than urging more overeating later. Whatever the mechanism, it is safe—and most likely particularly beneficial—to combine IF and exercise. A study from the Department of Kinesiology and Nutrition at the University of Illinois at Chicago found that obese subjects who combined alternate-day IF with an exercise program had better results than those who did only one of those interventions. They lost more weight and more fat, and also saw more improvement in blood cholesterol and lipid levels. That said, working out on IF may require a few tweaks to get maximum results.

### How and When: A Primer

First things first: Almost any form of exercise can be a match with your chosen plan. Whitaker is a big fan of walking, and also what he calls "wogging"—alternating between walking and jogging—and feels that some form of aerobic workout at a moderate intensity is crucial. He prescribes everything from running or wogging to cycling, swimming, stair-climbing, aerobics classes, playing racket sports or using an elliptical trainer. But stressing your muscles with weight training is important, too, and as you lose body fat your muscles will be more visible, says neuroscientist Mark Mattson, PhD. "It turns out that a lot of bodybuilders, perhaps by trial and error, have found that if they don't eat breakfast, work out midday or [when they're] around 16 hours fasted, and then eat later, they're able to maintain and build muscle while losing more

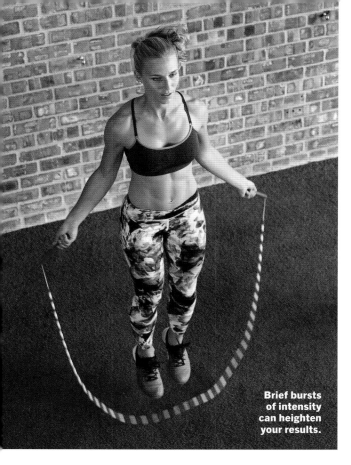

**Brief bursts of intensity can heighten your results.**

fat." Your best bet is a combination of aerobic and strength work on alternate days. Here's how to get started, and what to watch for.

**START SLOW** If you have been largely sedentary, begin with walking for 40 minutes a day, gradually increasing in speed and intensity, advises Whitaker. Even if you have already been athletic and active, you may notice a slowdown at first, says Jason Fung, MD, author of *The Complete Guide to Fasting*. "Exercising in the fasted state trains your muscles to burn fat, and they become much more efficient at doing that," says Fung. "But while you're adjusting to the change from burning sugar to burning fat—approximately two weeks—you may notice a temporary decrease in energy, muscle strength and overall exercise capacity." Consider reducing the weights you lift and cutting back your intensity for a couple of weeks. After that, you'll

find you actually have more endurance, because your muscles are better at using fat for fuel.

**LISTEN TO YOUR BODY** Learn to recognize what is normal you-can-push-through-it pain from working out and what is unusual for you, advises Jonathan Poyourow, RD, CSCS, a sports dietitian, professional chef and associate professor of nutrition at Johnson & Wales University. If it hurts in a bad way, stop doing it. Other things to look out for as you embark on a combined IF and exercise regimen: mental fog, insomnia, slow recovery from workouts, weakness or feelings of depression or burnout. IF isn't for everyone—or you may need to just cut back your effort until your fat-burning capacity catches up.

**TIME IT RIGHT** Depending on who you talk to, the best time to work out on IF is either right before you end your fast or several hours before you end it. Whitaker says he sees the best results when clients continue to fast after their workout, because "the longer the fasting period, the more efficient and prolonged the fat-burning is." You've probably depleted all your glycogen by the end of your workout, so every hour you fast after that is an hour of pure fat-burning. Other experts see particular benefits to chowing down right away. "A meal immediately after your workout will be stored most efficiently, mostly as glycogen for muscle stores, or burned as energy to help with the recovery process, and with minimal amounts stored as fat," says Ted Naiman, MD, co-author of *The P:E Diet*. Listen to your body: If you're ravenous after working out, there's nothing wrong with eating right away.

**EAT WELL** Since you'll be fueling a depleted body when you break your fast, it's especially important that you eat quality food, says Poyourow, who himself is a fan of the Mediterranean diet. "You need to make every meal count, nutrition-wise." That means healthy fats, protein, whole grains and fresh fruits and vegetables. "Why undo all your hard work in the gym by eating garbage?" Poyourow asks. "Go for the good stuff."

# A CLEANER
# PLATE

**Fasting by its very nature is a type of cleanse, allowing your body to devote all its energies to clearing out toxins. So why not amp up its powers even more?**

✕

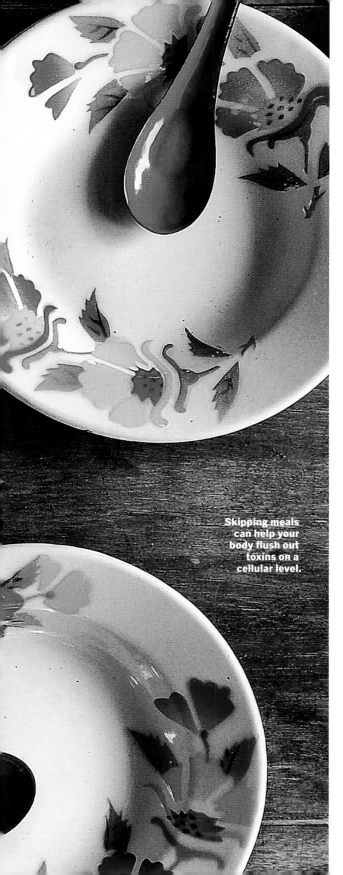

Skipping meals can help your body flush out toxins on a cellular level.

**CLEANSES ARE A** hot topic right now, and intermittent fasting fits perfectly into this desire to detoxify. Many cleanses can help jump-start weight loss, but there are also a number of benefits, including improvements in metabolism, insulin sensitivity, brain health and liver function. Fasting and cleansing work through similar pathways to make key changes in cells. When you combine the two plans, they boost health synergistically. That helps explain why many cleanses or detox regimens include fasting. It's also why both fasting and cleansing are ancient traditions long associated with spirituality and clarity. Consider how this dynamic duo works, and how to use cleansing to power up your fasting benefits.

## Reboot Your System

Both IF and cleansing effectively reset your entire system. IF's reboot is like what happens when you shut down your computer: When the demands of daily use are lowered, glitches and mistakes can be fixed and everything works better when it starts up again. "In a way, fasting is like changing the oil and transmission fluid in your car," says Peter Bennett, ND, co-author of *7-Day Detox Miracle*, whose detox plan starts with a two-day fast.

Most of the time, Bennett explains, your liver is super busy keeping your system clean and functioning efficiently, because it's your primary detoxifying organ. That's why, for instance, heavy drinkers can develop liver disease: Alcohol is a toxin, and too much of it can overtax the liver. Medications and food also pass through the liver. In essence, says Bennett, "The liver is a massive processing center that breaks down nutrients like fats and sugars from your foods, while also assembling molecules and hormone precursors, shifting energy into storage and cleaning the blood of the 'metabolic sweat' of every cell in your body." Imagine what happens when you take food out of the equation for a while. "The liver gets to play catch-up on all this assembling and disassembling, because it's not having to share time dealing with food. The longer you rest your liver from digestion, the cleaner your blood will be," Bennett says.

In a similar way, cleansing aims for a reboot by removing from your diet substances that stress your innate detoxification systems. These include things like sugar, alcohol and highly processed and nonorganic foods. Replacing them with nutrient- and fiber-rich whole foods reseeds your crucial gut microbiome. Cleanses also clear the way for your liver, lungs and lymph system to repair and rejuvenate by removing environmental toxins that come from chemicals, plastics, pollutants and pesticides.

## Calm Inflammation

Another key pathway that IF and cleansing share is their ability to reduce inflammation throughout the body. Inflammation has been linked to a long list of ailments, including heart disease, dementia, diabetes, arthritis and immune disorders. A recent study in the journal *Nature Medicine* found that diseases associated with chronic inflammation are "the most significant cause of death in the world today," causing more than 50 percent of deaths globally.

Fasting has been shown to lower systemic inflammation, perhaps in part due to the rebooting process. When you shut down the digestive process for a while, your body's natural healing abilities help clean up the debris from other processes of your body, a phenomenon called autophagy. Studies have shown that intermittent fasters have lower levels of C-reactive protein or CRP, a marker of inflammation.

Cleanses have a powerful effect on inflammation as well, because many of the items that are eliminated in a cleanse—processed foods and environmental toxins, for instance—are highly inflammatory. A single can of soda has been shown to increase inflammatory markers in the blood. In addition, a full cleansing program includes

other lifestyle elements, from stress reduction to better sleep, which also work to lower your levels of inflammation. The blueprint that follows will help you add cleansing elements to your IF program.

## Do a Mini-Cleanse

Many people picture a cleanse as a super-intense few days of existing only on juices, but modern cleansing is more sophisticated and well-rounded. Many pathways to detoxing your body have little to do with food—or juice. Add these cleansing actions to your IF lifestyle to help boost your fasting benefits:

GET BETTER SLUMBER Sleeping deeply for seven to nine hours a night is the easiest form of cleansing there is. Solid sack time detoxifies in part by helping your body, and especially your brain, reorganize and recharge itself. "It allows the brain to remove toxic waste byproducts that have accumulated throughout the day," says Gavin Van De Walle, MS, RD, president of Dakota Dietitians. This helps keep inflammation at bay. A study in the journal *Biological Psychiatry* found that just one bad night's sleep can trigger key cellular pathways that fuel inflammation.

Many studies have also found a link between inadequate slumber and weight gain, so if your goal is shedding pounds, go to bed! To boost your sleep hygiene, try these tips: Institute a

✕

## FASTING AND CLEANSING SHARE ANTI-INFLAMMATORY PATHWAYS, WHICH BOOSTS ORGAN HEALTH.

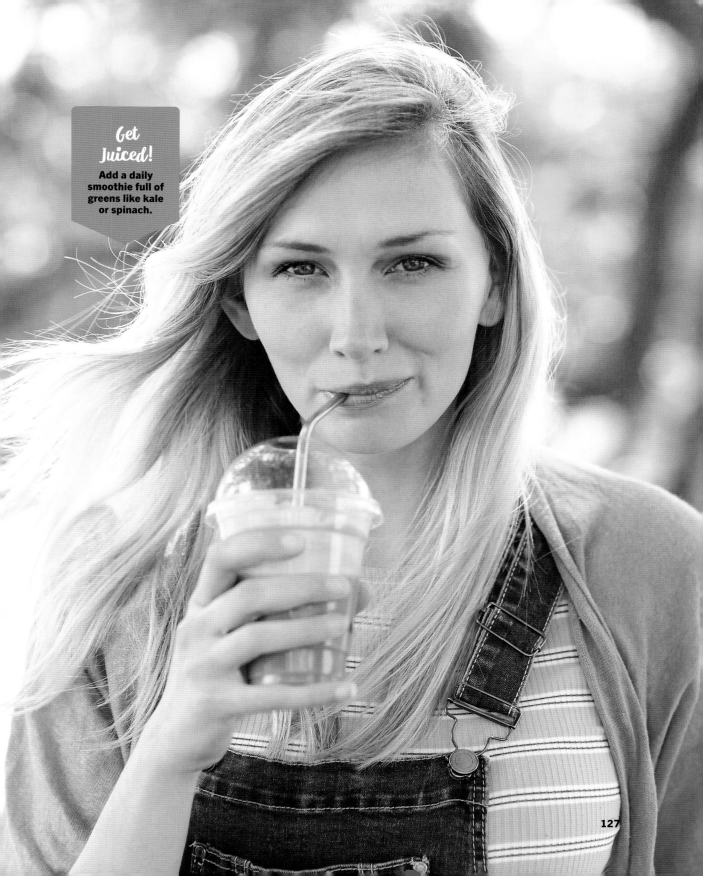

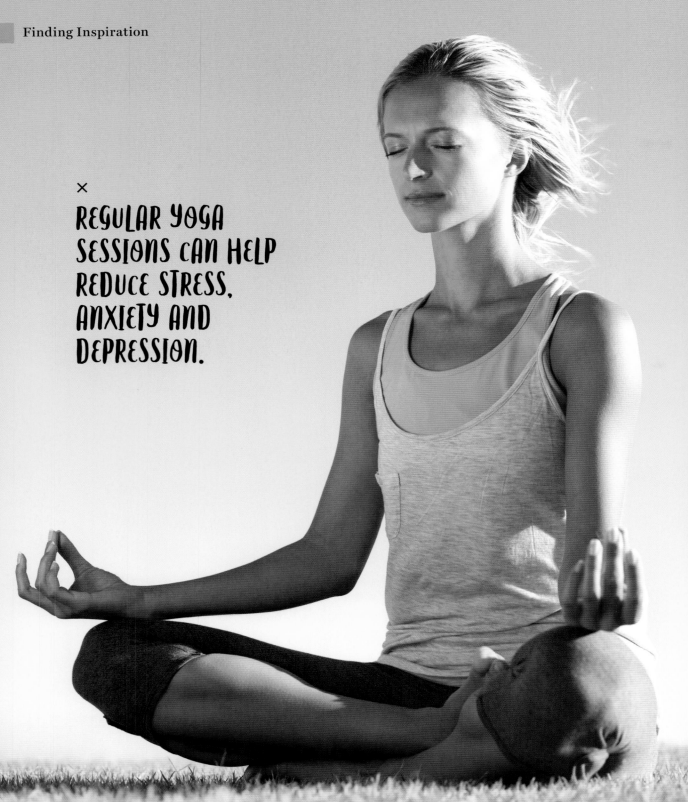

×

REGULAR YOGA
SESSIONS CAN HELP
REDUCE STRESS,
ANXIETY AND
DEPRESSION.

regular bedtime, put away blue-light sources (like computers or phones) two hours before lights-out time, cut down on coffee, and make sure your bedroom is cool and dark.

**REDUCE STRESS** It's more easily said than done, but there are many ways to start "unclenching" your mind and body. Two of the best are yoga and meditation. Studies have shown that practicing yoga can lower the secretion of cortisol, a stress hormone that is helpful for short-term pressures, but damaging if it lingers indefinitely. In addition, a study showed that people who did regular yoga sessions for 10 weeks had lower levels of inflammatory markers. You can get started with (often free) online classes, or try a few simple poses available via a quick Google search.

Meditation also has cleansing benefits. Like yoga, it lowers cortisol levels, and studies show it can aid blood pressure, help prevent cardiovascular disease and boost mental clarity. Check out free apps like Calm or Headspace.

**ELIMINATE SUGAR** Of all the dietary changes wrought by cleansing, perhaps the most important is eliminating added sugars (natural sugars in fruits and vegetables are fine). Sugar is endemic in our food supply, and evidence shows it can be highly addictive and inflammatory. "Sugar—along with processed foods—is thought to be at the root of today's public health crises," says Van De Walle. Sugar hinders your body's ability to detoxify itself by harming key detoxing organs like the liver. It is also a culprit in diabetes and heart disease, due to its inflammatory properties. The best way to reduce added sugars is to avoid processed and fast foods. Even foods that don't taste sweet, like crackers, are often loaded with sugar.

**MAKE BROTH** Bone broth (or vegetable broth if you're vegan) has a place of honor in cleansing, because it has a powerful effect on your microbiome, which is essential to digestive and immune health. Plus, broth is a mainstay when you're doing alternate-day fasting or an extended fast of a day or two. (See page 116 for recipe.)

## Instant Cleansing
### Want to jump-start your fasting cleanse?
### Try these moves:

**SWEAT**
Whether it's from exercise or a sauna session, sweating helps usher toxins out of your system through one of your most important cleansing pathways: your skin. Just be sure to drink lots of water afterward.

**DO A DEVICE DETOX**
Being constantly connected to news and chatter is detrimental to your mental health and sense of calm. Designate specific periods when you'll turn off the screens and simply focus on the world around you.

**CLEAN HOUSE**
Buy some green cleaning products and do a full sweep of your dwelling. Studies show that indoors can be more polluted than outdoors, due to chemical residue from cleaning and personal-health items as well as flame retardants and other problematic chemicals like endocrine disrupters. Look for a vacuum cleaner with a HEPA filter to pick up the smallest particles in your home.

**DRINK UP**
Water itself is cleansing, and is also key to fasting. Keep a glass or bottle of water at your side all day and keep sipping.

**SHOP ORGANIC**
This is an easy way to start clearing your body of toxins like pesticides and fungicides. Also look for grass-fed, pasture-raised beef, chicken and eggs.

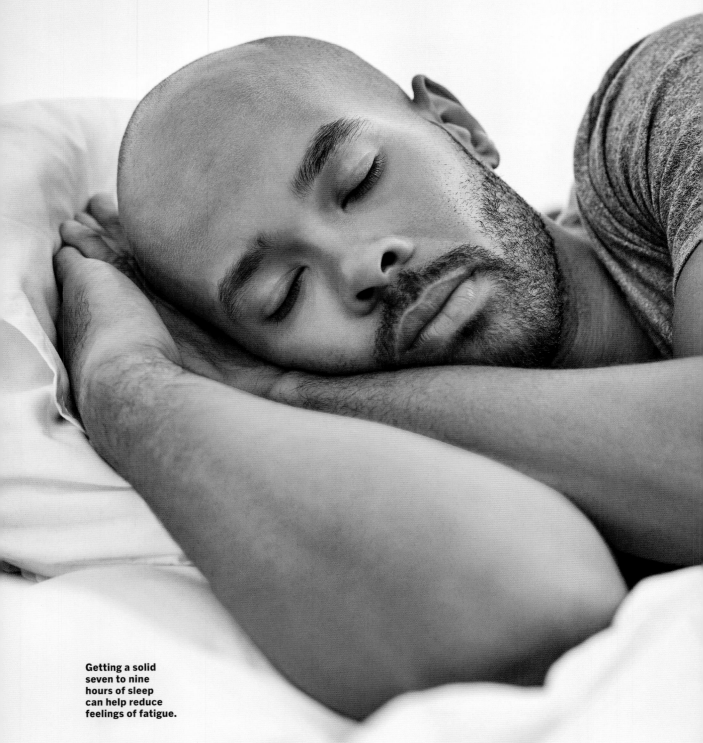

**Getting a solid
seven to nine
hours of sleep
can help reduce
feelings of fatigue.**

# SKIP THE
# SIDE EFFECTS

**The good news: There aren't very many of them.
When they do crop up, try these strategies.**

**CHANGING THE WAY** you eat has its challenges. But the intriguing thing about intermittent fasting is that evidence is increasingly showing two things: These perceived obstacles are no greater than those of "regular" dieting (daily calorie restriction), and they subside over time. "Feeling hungry and irritable is common initially, and usually passes after two weeks to a month as the body and brain become accustomed to the new habit," says Mark Mattson, PhD, a professor of neuroscience at Johns Hopkins University, who has studied IF for 25 years (and has followed a time-restricted plan himself for decades).

Mattson feels that even these side effects can be greatly mitigated by easing into an IF program rather than going at it full bore. He recommends, for instance, that someone starting a 16:8 plan begin with a 10-hour feeding period (14:10) five days a week for a month. Only then does he suggest

going down to a 16:8 plan, still for five days a week, for the second month, before proceeding to 16:8 daily—or even moving slowly toward a daily six-hour feeding period (18:6), which is what Mattson follows. For 5:2 fasters, he says, begin with one 1,000-calorie day per week for a month, then up it to two days a week, slowly reducing calories for fasting days to 750, then 500. This gives your system time to learn how to access body fat for fuel.

One key point that virtually all IF studies find is that "no major adverse effects were reported." For any other minor complaints of newbie fasters, try these quick fixes.

## Headaches

These are likely due to a drop in salt intake, says Megan Ramos, co-founder and program director of the Intensive Dietary Management Program. "This is the No. 1 cause of almost all of the physical side effects of fasting, from headaches to gout attacks," says Ramos. That's because while fasting, you're not consuming the foods that normally keep your salt levels up, and sodium is essential to your body. Ramos suggests consuming bone broth with added salt, or sugar-free pickle juice. Mineral water is another source. In addition, says Ramos, "Be more generous with your salt intake on your eating days when seasoning food." She adds one caveat: "Check with your doctor—people who have chronic kidney disease or certain cardiovascular conditions need to be mindful of their sodium intake."

## Fatigue

Some people feel a dip in energy when starting a fasting regimen, although the numbers aren't large—for instance, only 8 percent of subjects

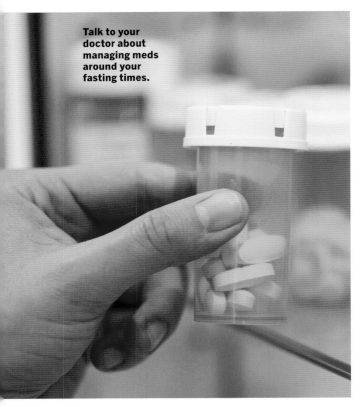

**Talk to your doctor about managing meds around your fasting times.**

✕

# CAFFEINE WITHDRAWAL CAN ALSO TRIGGER HEADACHES; BLACK COFFEE OR TEA CAN HELP.

in a study published in the *British Journal of Nutrition* complained of fatigue, and 6 percent in the same study said they felt an *increase* in energy. If you do start dragging, says Ramos, the worst thing you can do is take it easy. What's probably happening, she explains, is that your body is running low on easily accessed fuel from glycogen, and it hasn't taken the next step of breaking down body fat for fuel. Basically, it needs a nudge. "If you continue to fast and also slightly increase energy demands, you'll force your body to start burning body fat and refueling your system," says Ramos. You don't need a major workout; just move your muscles by walking. Sounds counterintuitive, but it's true.

## Dizziness

Feeling lightheaded is not a super-common problem, but if you do experience it, up your intake of both salt and water—it's likely a simple matter of dehydration. If you're on blood pressure meds, though, consult your physician to make sure your BP isn't going too low.

## Constipation

Hydration is, again, a huge help with bowel issues. In fact, dehydration is key to so many side effects of fasting that "you may need to set a reminder on your phone to alert you to drink every couple of hours throughout the day," says Ramos. Increasing your intake of fiber, fruits and vegetables during your feeding times can also help get things moving again.

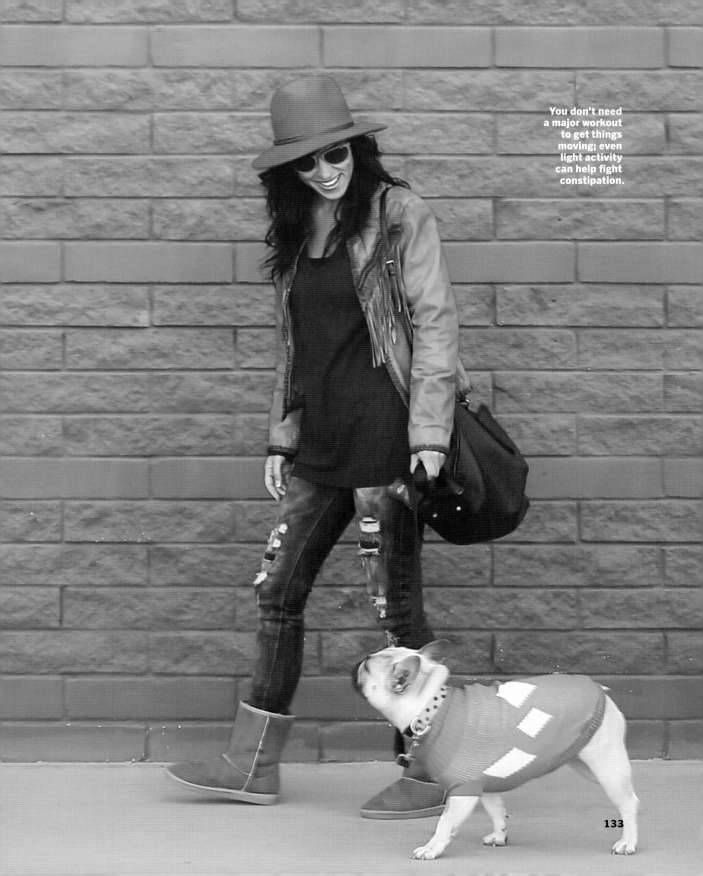

You don't need a major workout to get things moving; even light activity can help fight constipation.

133

# THE FASTING LIFESTYLE

INSIGHT, ADVICE AND
PERSPECTIVE FOR CHARTING
YOUR NEW COURSE.

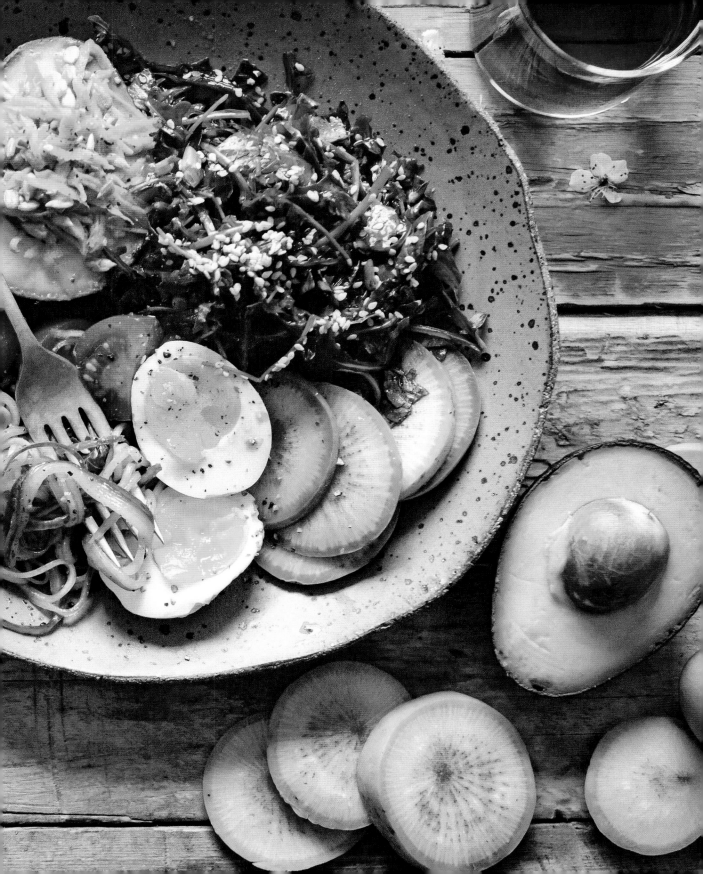

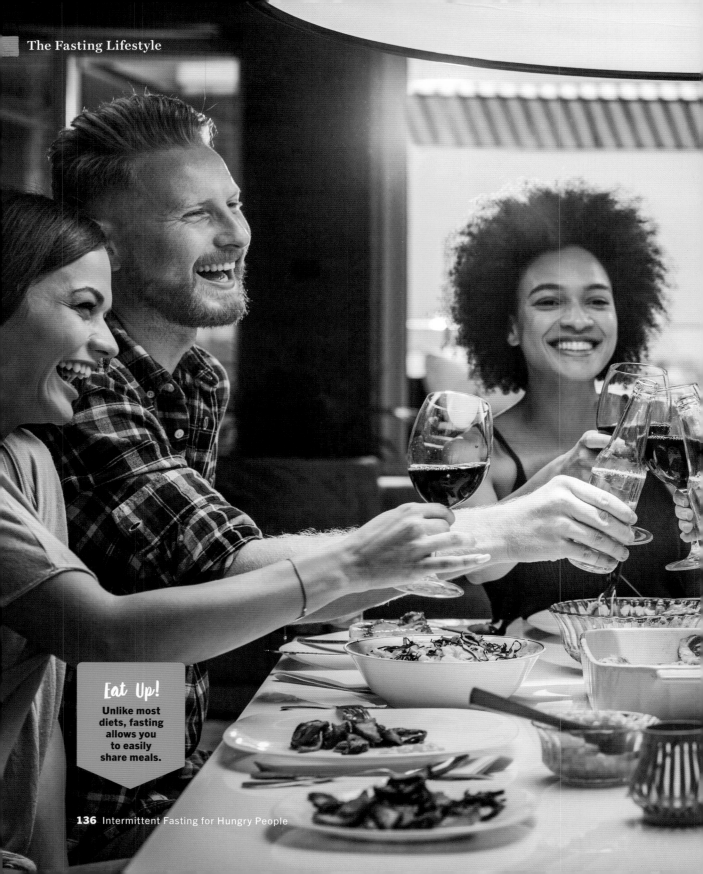

### Eat Up!

Unlike most diets, fasting allows you to easily share meals.

# GO THE
# DISTANCE

**Four key techniques for the
long haul, from breaking bad habits
to recovering from slipups.**

×

**NOBODY'S PERFECT. THAT'S** a good thing to keep in mind if you want your fasting program to become a lasting romance rather than a brief fling. There will be times when the demands of your particular plan will hit roadblocks: a super-stressful day, an unexpected night out or simple fasting fatigue. But one of the beauties of intermittent fasting is its flexibility: It is almost infinitely malleable, so if an impediment springs up here, you can circumvent it there. Here's how to sail through IF crises on cruise control.

## Make It Social

That means both keeping up your social life and sharing the benefits of your fasting experiences with others. IF is actually one of the easiest diet programs to stick to while still enjoying nights out and dinner parties, because you can adjust your fasting window or fasting days to accommodate special events—or even just family dinners. For instance, Kristin Hoddy, PhD, RDN, a researcher who has studied fasting (and incorporated it into her own life), describes how she experimented with ways to work it into her schedule. When she was trying out the 5:2 plan, she switched from having one midday meal into two smaller ones: that way, she could sit down to dinner with her husband.

"The nice thing about alternate-day or 5:2 fasting is that you don't have to worry about 'dieting' on your feast days—you can socialize and eat normally," says Krista Varady, PhD, a professor of nutrition at the University of Illinois at Chicago, and author of *The Every Other Day Diet*. And with time-restricted plans like 16:8, all you need to do to maintain a social life is position your eating window for when you want to go out, whether for a lunch date or for dinner. "As clinicians, we have to realize that people need to follow a plan they can incorporate into their lifestyle, that mimics the way they already live," Varady says. Intermittent fasting offers the flexibility to do exactly that.

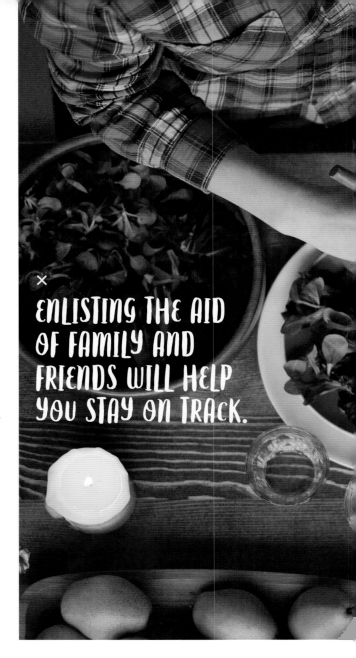

ENLISTING THE AID OF FAMILY AND FRIENDS WILL HELP YOU STAY ON TRACK.

As far as the other meaning of "social," many fasters find that sharing their experiences via social media helps energize them to stick with the program—witness the huge rise in Instagram tags related to IF, which now number in the millions. Posting your progress on Instagram or Facebook

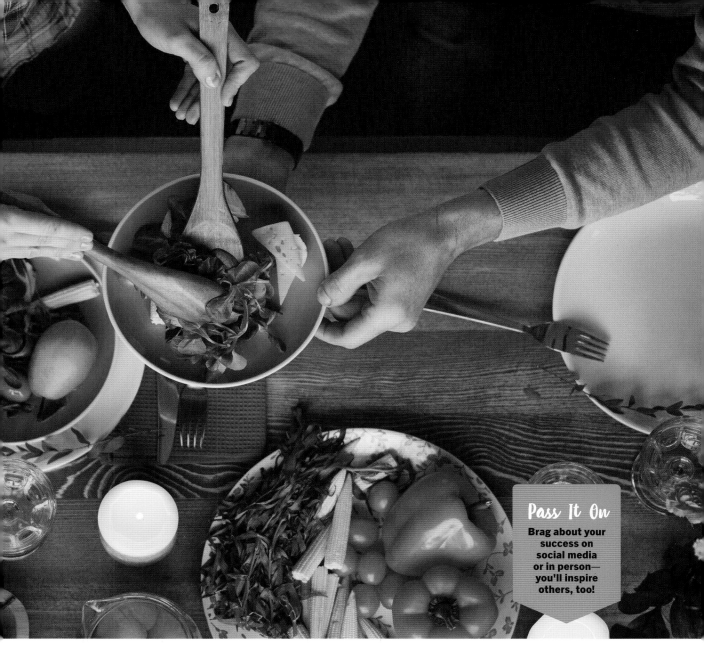

makes it seem more "real," and being cheered on by friends and followers is highly motivating. Be sure to take a "before" photo!

## Rethink Your Habits

Much of our eating is habitual, like Pavlov's dogs who salivated when they saw attendants in white coats: They associated the coats with being fed.

We look up from our desks at noon or 1 p.m. and think, "Time to eat."

"Seeing the clock hit midday is your cue that it's break time," says Megan Ramos, co-founder of the Intensive Dietary Management Program. "For years you've taken the action of eating lunch to get that break, but it's worth asking yourself if you're actually hungry, or whether you just need

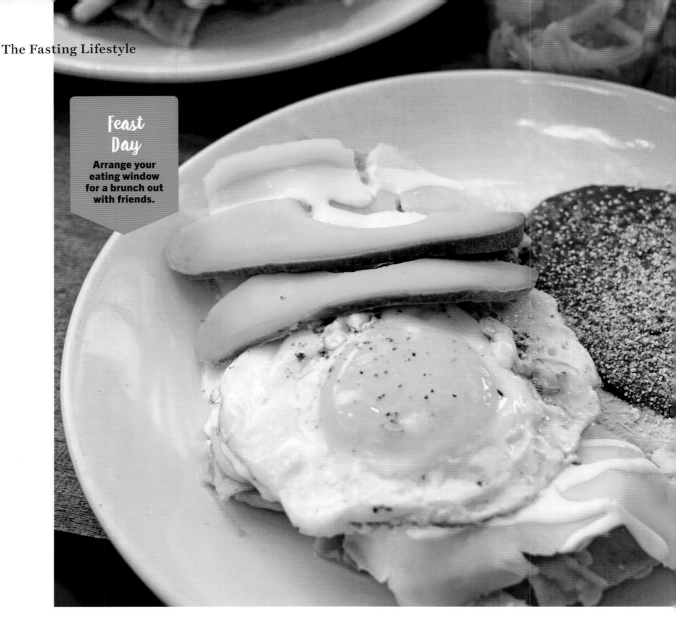

**Feast Day**

Arrange your eating window for a brunch out with friends.

a break. If it's the latter, you could grab a coffee or tea and go for a walk, read a book or listen to a podcast. You could even meditate." All of those can make you feel more refreshed and focused than wolfing down lunch at your desk.

Similarly, it's a natural human impulse to use an eating occasion as the time to catch up with friends or family—but it's not inevitable. "Humans have been socializing and building communities around feasting since the beginning of time," says Ramos. "But the truth is, there are many ways to connect with loved ones." If you're at home with kids, you can play a game, put together a puzzle or head outside for a walk. If you're planning a get-together with a friend, it doesn't have to be lunch, cocktails or dinner—you could go for a hike, take in a concert or check out an art exhibit at a local museum. It's freeing, and often enriching, to separate out eating from other activities.

# BOREDOM IS THE ACHILLES' HEEL OF MANY DIET PLANS, BUT FASTING LEAVES ROOM FOR VARIATION.

## Forgive Yourself

Were you too ravenous this morning to wait until noon or 1 p.m. before breaking your fast? Did you eat more than 500 to 600 calories on a fasting day? Remember, one of the best things about IF is its flexibility—and feeling guilty is counterproductive. "If you planned on fasting 16 hours but only make it to 13, that's OK," says Ted Naiman, MD, co-author of *The P:E Diet*. "You're still much better off than if you had eaten all day long, with early and late calories plus lots of snacking. Anything beyond a 12-hour window is going to be at least somewhat beneficial toward your goals. So fast for as long as is convenient, and break your fast whenever you need to or want to."

Naiman counts hours of fasting per week—additional to a baseline of 12:12—rather than keeping to a rigid schedule. "A good goal is 24 hours a week of extra fasting," Naiman says. This could be two days a week of 24-hour fasting (5:2), three days of eight-hour fasting (OMAD/Warrior), or six days of four-hour fasting (16:8). So if, say, you "screwed up" one of your 16:8 days, you could fast a few extra hours the following day. As Naiman says, it's all good.

## Change It Up

Along the same lines, "surprising" your system with a change in schedule or in the types of food

you're eating can also help keep things interesting and on track. Naiman suggests a mix-and-match approach in general: "All of these different fasting methods are effective, and I recommend keeping it flexible." Your body may even benefit from the change, in the same way that "muscle confusion"—changing up your exercise routine to work different muscles—can improve your strength and fitness.

One way to do this is to throw a full-day fast into the mix, or add a couple of OMAD days to a week of 16:8 days. But you could also cycle in some days of low-carb or keto eating, which can work as a jump-start of sorts. You don't need to be in continuous dietary ketosis to reap extra benefits from keto. Just try planning a day, or several days, of low-carb meals. That means focusing on fats, protein and non-starchy vegetables, and nixing the grains. (See page 84 for more details.)

---

### Secret Weapons
Put these in your arsenal to help you stay the course.

**CINNAMON**
This delicious spice has been shown to slow gastric emptying and may help suppress hunger and lower blood-sugar levels. Add some to your tea or coffee.

**GREEN TEA**
Not only does it have antioxidants and polyphenols that confer all kinds of health benefits, but it's an appetite suppressant.

**CHIA SEEDS**
Super high in soluble fiber and omega-3 fatty acids, these absorb water and form a gel or pudding when soaked for 30 minutes. Although technically breaking the fast, experts say the hunger suppression effects more than make up for the minimal calories.

**STAR ANISE**
This spice can help calm an upset stomach.

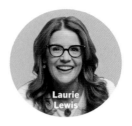

# ADVICE

## FROM A PRO

**Laurie Lewis isn't just a personal IF success story—
she helps other people reach their goals. Here's her
hard-won wisdom on how to make IF work for you.**

**ONE NIGHT IN** 2012, Laurie Lewis did what any
woman going through menopause—and depressed
over how it was holding her body hostage—might
do: She went Googling for solutions. "I crawled
into bed with my laptop and Googled 'hormonal,
menopausal, stubborn fat' and up popped a
YouTube video about intermittent fasting—and
then another and another," she says.

"I stayed up all night watching videos. I had no
idea you should live your life pausing from eating
every day." Or that doing so would not only help her
shed the 50 pounds she'd gained, but set her on a
wellness journey that would transform her life. "I'd
been a runner and a super-healthy eater for over 20
years," says Lewis. "Everyone was, like, 'How could

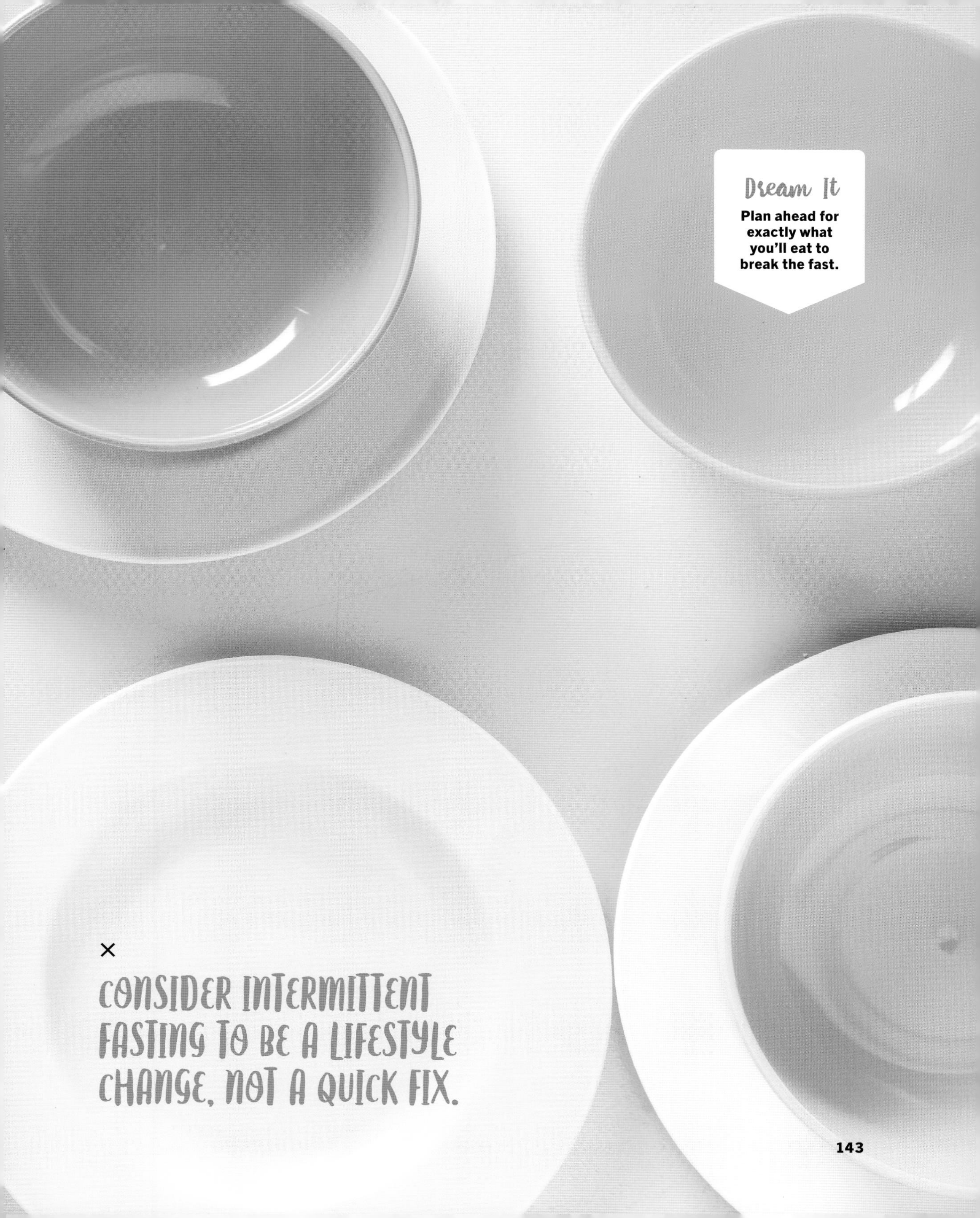

**Dream It**

Plan ahead for exactly what you'll eat to break the fast.

✕

# CONSIDER INTERMITTENT FASTING TO BE A LIFESTYLE CHANGE, NOT A QUICK FIX.

you gain 50 pounds? You're the healthiest person we know.' But it was less about what I looked like and more about how I felt. I felt like an alien had taken over my body. And nothing I did turned it around." Until she tried intermittent fasting.

Now an integrative nutrition coach based in Portland, Oregon, Lewis helps others iron out the wrinkles in their fasting experience through workshops and one-on-one sessions. Here, she addresses the ups and downs you can expect from life in the fasting lane.

**Q** **What's your best piece of advice for someone just starting off with IF?**

Take it one fast and one feast at a time. So many people who are new to fasting want to be told precisely what to do. I tell them: "It's simple. You just stop eating for a certain amount of hours and you fast clean." But what I've learned is that in the first two to four weeks, people really want to be told exactly what to do every day. So the thing about listening to your body? That comes later. In the beginning, people are, like, "If I listen to my body I'll eat cupcakes!" Another thing I tell people new to fasting: "Don't try to change everything at

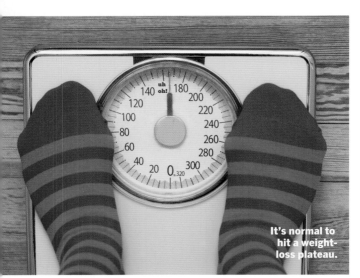

It's normal to hit a weight-loss plateau.

# GIVE YOURSELF TIME TO CHOOSE YOUR PLAN. IT TOOK LEWIS SEVERAL TRIES TO MASTER ALTERNATE-DAY.

once." Going hours without eating is a feat! Get used to practicing intermittent fasting every day, and then your body will tell you when it's time to start the other stuff—like, for instance, beginning a new exercise regimen.

**Q** **How do you know which approach is best for you?**

Start by keeping it simple. Think about it this way: There are two parts to every day, the fasting part and the eating part. On the first day, you'll decide what time you're going to stop eating. Then you'll go to bed, wake up, and eat 12 hours after you stopped eating. Then you'll decide if you're a rip-the-bandage-off kind of person and fast for 16 hours the next day. Or do you want to gradually increase your fasting period by 15 minutes every day? In the beginning, it's important to pencil in when you're going to fast, what your window will be and what delicious foods you're going to eat. Knowing the foods you're going to eat is extremely motivating. After about two weeks, try a stretch and see if you can go to 18 hours.

**Q** **Many people shy away from intermittent fasting because they're afraid they'll go hungry. How do you get through the hunger pangs?**

I call them "hunger waves." People need to know that hunger doesn't build and build; it comes in a wave. We think stomach grumblings mean we're

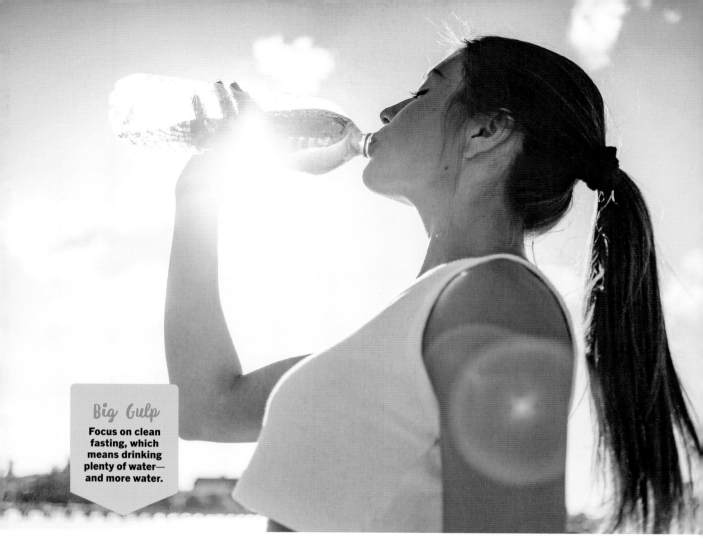

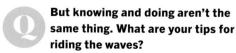

**Big Gulp**

**Focus on clean fasting, which means drinking plenty of water— and more water.**

dying of starvation, but it doesn't mean that. We have to get through the discomfort by knowing it's temporary, and by keeping in mind the motivation. For me, what was motivating was knowing what was happening to my body. I became deeply committed to keeping insulin low, burning stored body fat for fuel, and ramping up the cellular repair process called autophagy. For all of that to happen, I knew that I had to keep going.

**Q But knowing and doing aren't the same thing. What are your tips for riding the waves?**

You can either get really busy to distract yourself and do something wonderful and fun.

Or do the opposite and sit mindfully, breathe into it and do nothing. That hunger wave will subside.

**Q You've said that the second month of IF tends to be a turning point. How so?**

The second month is when people get really impatient and they either quit—even though they've never felt better in their lives—or, on the plus side, they get into a fasting groove. That's when it's time to take a close look at your eating window: What are you eating to open your window and break your fast? What's the pace at which you're eating? Are you trying to squeeze two complete meals into a five-hour eating window where one meal spread out over a few hours and

**145**

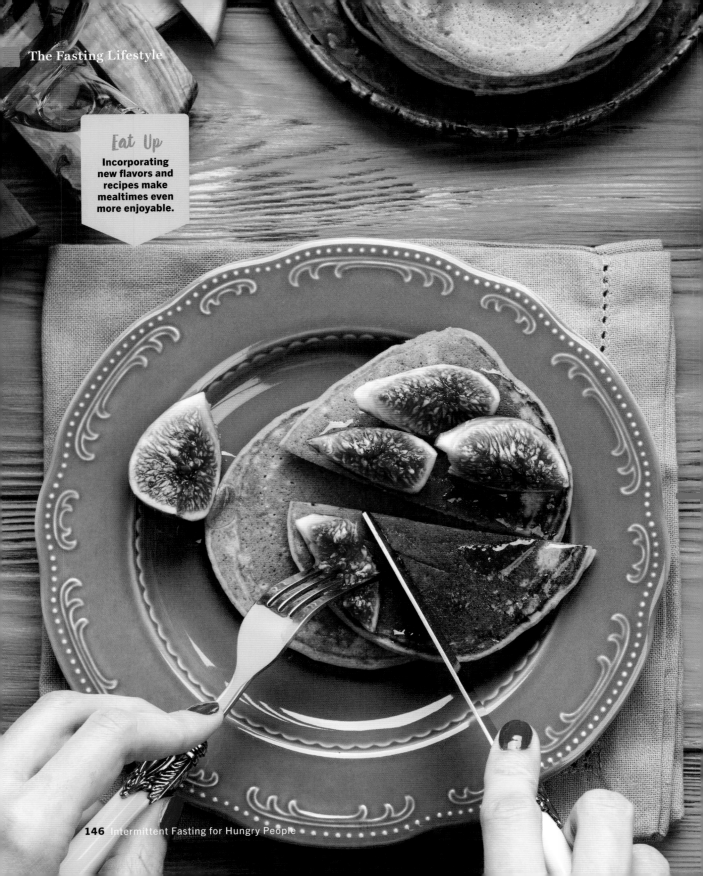

**Eat Up**

Incorporating new flavors and recipes make mealtimes even more enjoyable.

# KEEPING A JOURNAL WHEN YOU'RE STARTING OUT CAN HELP YOU FIGURE OUT WHAT WORKS AND BOOST MOTIVATION.

a snack would be sufficient? That investigation happens in the second month, either naturally in a conversation with a coach or through journaling.

**Q Speaking of turning points: How do you get past a plateau?**

Switch it up! I started with 16:8, moved to 18:6, then stayed on a 20:4 plan after six weeks. After nine months, I'd lost a pound or two per week on average. But then I stalled—for five months. Someone encouraged me to try alternate-day fasting, which is a 36- to 40-hour fast with an eight- to 12-hour eating window. On the second day, I thought, "I'm so used to eating every 20 hours I just want to eat!" So it took a few tries to get me over the hump. And I really had to make sure that on the day I was eating, I was eating a lot—getting two meals in an eight-hour window—and listening to my body. We know to eat to satiety with any plan, but that's especially true if you take on alternate-day fasting. On my "regular days," I had a big long window and two full chow-down meals. Then I would do a day of almost total fasting. Switching things up worked. Within a few months I had lost 51 pounds.

**Q What's the No.1 way people trip themselves up?**

They don't fast "clean." They add cream to their coffee, or they drink tea with cloves, ginger, orange flavoring or lemongrass, not

realizing how it can sabotage results. All of those flavors inform the body that food is incoming, and then the body prepares hormonally for the digestion process. Two reasons we don't want to bring those flavors in: First, it makes fasting a lot harder. And secondly, it stops the fat-burning process. During the fasting hours, you should fast clean, clean, clean—squeaky clean!—then have whatever you want in your eating window.

**Q What are some other tricks to get over stuck points?**

Setting the right mindset really helps. When I was starting out, I researched the very best mineral water with the greatest mineral content. And I would look forward to having a big, tall, icy glass of sparkling mineral water at 2 or 3 in the afternoon. If my stomach was growling—which it still does every day—I would tell myself: "Your body is trying to get you to feed it before it switches over to fat-burning, so just let it growl." Then I'd thank my body for burning fat and tell it to just keep grumbling away like it's a fat-burning furnace.

**Q What's the secret to staying motivated, especially during the periods when the scale doesn't budge?**

Keep thinking empowering thoughts. It doesn't have to be some elaborate fasting mantra. It can be as simple as: "I know this is good for me" or "This makes me happy" or "My body is amazing." Whatever motivates you. If getting into your skinny jeans motivates you, great! Keep them in a prominent location so that if you want to eat at 10 a.m. and your goal is to fast until noon, you can look at those skinny jeans.

**Q What do all successful intermittent fasters have in common?**

They are supremely patient. I tell my clients all the time: "Give yourself a year. Do not give yourself an out."

# THE
# SETBACK
# SOLUTION

### Here, eight ways to blast past stuck points and conquer cravings.

**NO MATTER HOW** motivated you are, you're sure to encounter some roadblocks and tricky situations as you smooth the way to an intermittent fasting routine. The moments when everyone is snacking and munching, except you. That time of day when you're accustomed to devouring a bagel or muffin on the way to work. The late-night cravings for a big piece of cake—long after your eating window has closed for the day. To the rescue: These eight tried-and-true methods can help you power through and keep you on track for success.

### 1 Stay Busy

When it comes to fasting, distraction is the better part of valor. The biggest mistake you could make is to treat a fast day like a "day off" or low-activity day. Study after study shows that most people feel sharper, rather than duller, as they go through a fast. So use that brain power to get a lot done while also keeping your mind off the vending machine. And make new plans for your danger times by, say, replacing happy hour with the gym.

### 2 Give It 15 Minutes

Hunger comes in waves, says Michael Mosley, MD, author of *The Fast Diet*. "The idea is to put food in its place," Mosley explains. "It's only food. And hunger naturally subsides. Once you start to think about food in a rational and realistic way, you'll discover that you can modify your behavior around it. You can even push it aside." A bonus, he says, is that you start to become much more attuned to your body, with a keener sensitivity to appetite, hunger and satiety (which can change from day to day). If you still feel ravenous after 15 minutes or so, then you can think about whether you truly need to break your fast with some real food—or just settle your stomach with a cup of herbal tea.

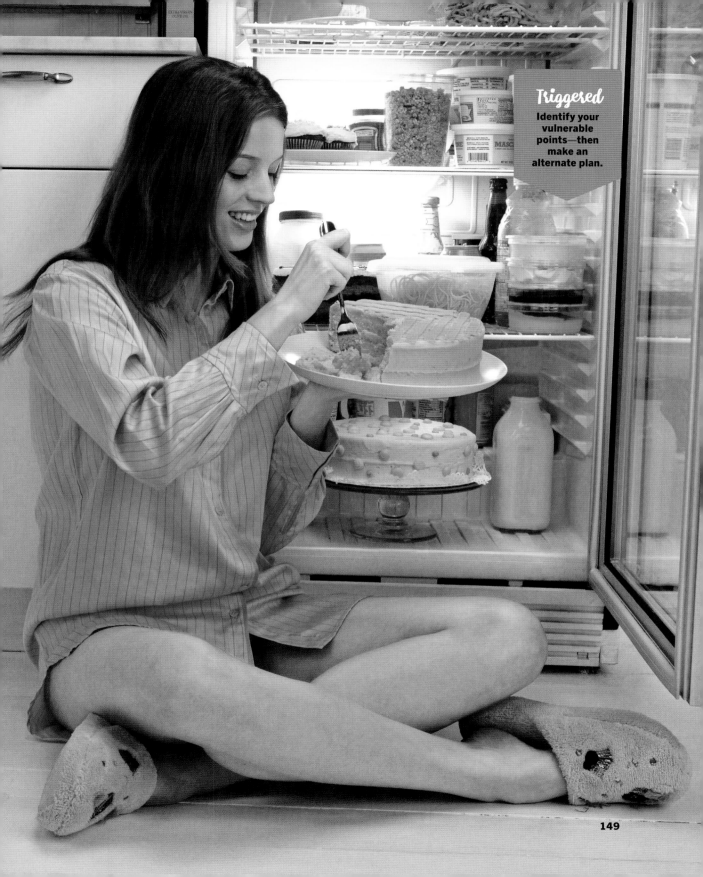

**Your Weak Spot?**

If certain foods make you overdo it, find a tasty substitute.

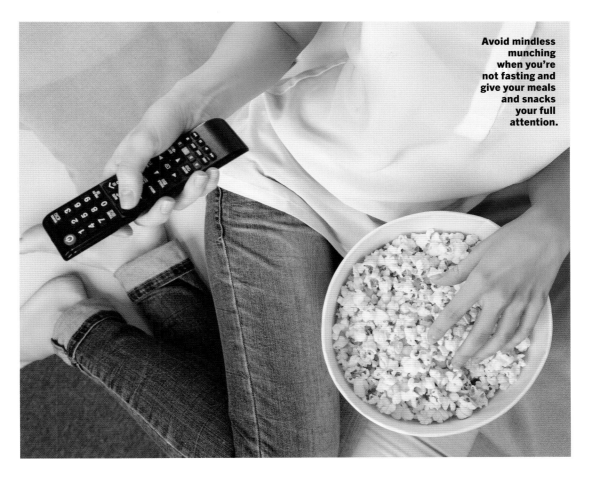

Avoid mindless munching when you're not fasting and give your meals and snacks your full attention.

### 3 ...And Give It a Month

Make a simple commitment to stick with an IF plan for four weeks, advises Jason Fung, MD, co-founder of the Intensive Dietary Management Program in Toronto. "It takes time for your body to get used to fasting," Fung explains. "Don't be discouraged. It gets easier." It also will take a little time to see results, so if you quit after a week or two you'll never know how much progress you might have made. If one type of fasting isn't working for you—alternate-day or 5:2 seem too challenging, for instance—switch to another form, like time-restricted 16:8, and see if that fasting schedule is more to your liking.

### 4 Think About Your Food

Yes, it does sound counterintuitive, but remember that saying "Try not to think of a pink elephant?" It's been shown that when you try to suppress certain thoughts, they're actually more likely to intrude, a phenomenon known as the "ironic process theory." The harder you try not to think of a pink elephant (or a lovely lunch), the more those images will present themselves. And not only will your efforts at suppression be in vain, but research shows that when it comes to food, indulging in delicious thoughts may be helpful. A study in the journal *Science* found that people who were told to repeatedly imagine eating a particular food, such as cheese, later ate less of that food compared to those who had only imagined eating it a few times, who imagined eating a different food (such as candy), or who didn't imagine eating at all. And they ate less of it simply because their desire was less pressing, not because it seemed unpalatable. This may be because of a process called "habituation"— after you've eaten, say, a hamburger, you're less interested in hamburgers. The amazing part is that you can become habituated just through your imagination. So go on and let visions of burgers and fries dance in your head during a fast.

### 5 Track Your Progress

Keeping an eye on improvements in your health and weight can be hugely motivating. Studies have shown that regular weigh-ins—whether you decide that should be every day, every few days or weekly—are associated with more weight loss than weigh-ins every month or longer. "Avoid fixating on the numbers on the scale, though, especially at first," advises Julian Whitaker, MD, founder of the Whitaker Wellness Institute. That's because, particularly if you are exercising, you may be replacing fat with muscle, "which may not show up right away as pounds lost." Whitaker recommends using your waist-to-hip ratio (see box on page 154) as a better marker, for two reasons: Abdominal fat is a serious health risk (called visceral fat, it wraps around your organs and releases toxins and disruptive hormones into

✕

## INADEQUATE SLEEP CAN CREATE HORMONAL CHANGES THAT LEAD TO MORE HUNGER PANGS.

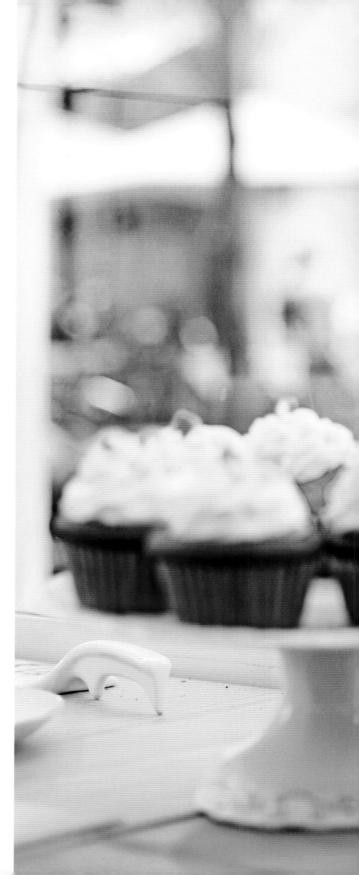

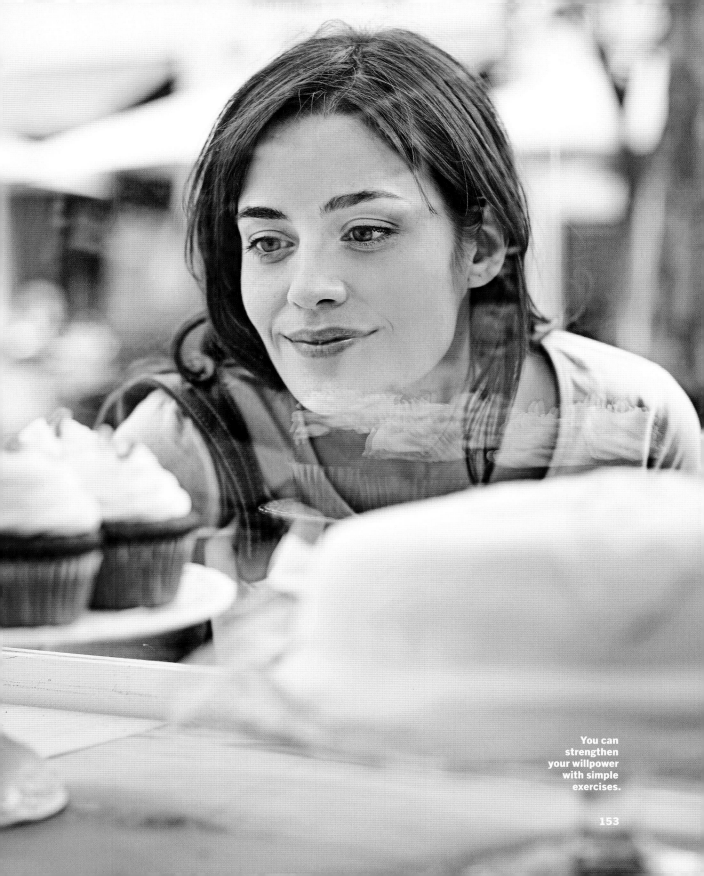

You can strengthen your willpower with simple exercises.

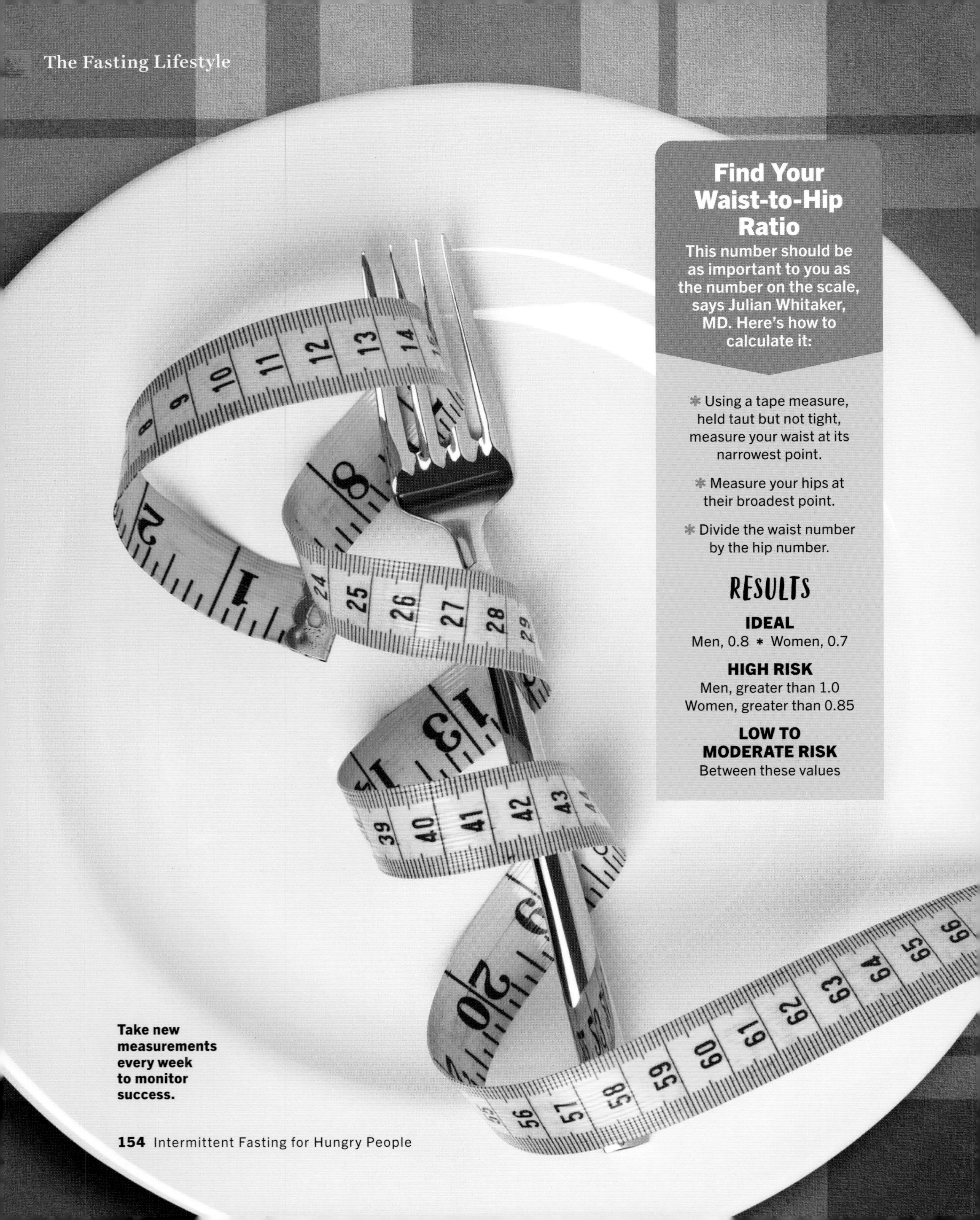

## Find Your Waist-to-Hip Ratio

This number should be as important to you as the number on the scale, says Julian Whitaker, MD. Here's how to calculate it:

* Using a tape measure, held taut but not tight, measure your waist at its narrowest point.

* Measure your hips at their broadest point.

* Divide the waist number by the hip number.

### RESULTS

**IDEAL**
Men, 0.8 * Women, 0.7

**HIGH RISK**
Men, greater than 1.0
Women, greater than 0.85

**LOW TO MODERATE RISK**
Between these values

**Take new measurements every week to monitor success.**

your system); and because it's very metabolically active, it's also the first fat to be mobilized and burned off when you start a fasting regimen. You're likely to see improvements in your measurements more quickly than on the scale, so keep a chart of the changes in both—and celebrate your progress along the way.

### 6 Prioritize Sleep

Numerous studies have shown that sleep and weight are intimately linked, with the rise in obesity over the past 50 years coinciding with the decline in the number of hours spent sleeping. On average, the less people sleep, the more they weigh, according to the National Sleep Foundation. The cutoff appears to be about seven hours; below that, you're sleep-deprived, although the ideal is between seven and nine. Imaging studies suggest that when you're sleep-deprived, your brain responds differently to unhealthy foods, making them more tempting. Not getting enough sleep also lowers your metabolic rate and throws various hormones out of whack, including insulin, ghrelin (which increases appetite) and leptin (the satiety hormone). Think of a good eight hours as part of your fasting regimen, and promote it by turning off any screens at least an hour before bedtime, and keeping your bedroom dark and cool. And remember: While you're snoozing, you're also fasting!

### 7 Exercise Your Willpower

Really, "exercise" it. Roy Baumeister, PhD, a professor at Florida State University, has studied willpower extensively and found that it operates much like a muscle. It can get fatigued with overuse, but it can also become stronger. This has led to two ideas about willpower: You can avoid overuse by "conserving" it, and you can strengthen it with small exercises. In a study in the *Journal of Personality and Social Psychology*, Baumeister found that making detailed plans— for instance, turning some of your difficult tasks

**✕**

## DON'T GET OBSESSED WITH NUMBERS—LOOK AT CHANGES THAT OCCUR OVER WEEKS, NOT DAYS.

into a habit, like packing a lunch for work rather than winging it at the salad bar—improves your odds for success. "Habits do not actually increase willpower; they conserve it," says Baumeister. Other studies have found that committing to any small, consistent act of self-control, whether it's keeping track of your spending or even saying "yes" instead of "yeah," increases overall willpower. "Through each of these willpower exercises, the brain gets used to pausing before acting," explains Kelly McGonigal, PhD, author of *The Willpower Instinct*. Translation for intermittent fasters: Set up guidelines and rules for your fasts so you don't have to constantly "use" your willpower to control yourself (pre-planning your meals on 5:2; making a list of allowed beverages during the fasting window on 16:8). And practice willpower on small, attainable tasks unrelated to fasting (getting up a half-hour earlier; avoiding swearing).

### 8 Know Your Triggers

It's estimated that people in today's food-infused culture make more than 200 eating decisions a day. Inevitably, some of those will be challenging, but everyone has his or her own personal food triggers that can threaten to wreak havoc on even the best-laid plans. Reflect on yours, and how to cut them off before the temptation bell rings, advises Mosley. "Try to instill a behavior that alters your established route," he says. If you know you're a late-night forager at home, for instance, circumvent the head-in-the-fridge moment by taking a relaxing bath.

# BOOST
## YOUR PLAN

**Dietary supplements—along with any medications you're already taking—require extra attention when you are following a fast.**

**PILLS OF ANY** kind are an interesting proposition on a fasting program. Various supplements can be a contributor to your overall wellness, filling in any nutritional gaps you may encounter as you change your eating patterns. And yet supplements, as well as any prescription meds you may be taking, can be dicey on an empty stomach. Not only that, but as your health status changes due to an intermittent fasting plan—if you have high blood pressure it may go down; if you have diabetes, your blood sugar status may improve— you may well need a change in your prescription. Read on for a breakdown of how to deal with pills of all kinds as you embark on IF.

## Supplements: Yes or No?

First, some perspective. It's unlikely that anyone in America today, at least if they're living above the poverty line, will suffer from diseases of vitamin deficiency like rickets, anemia or scurvy.

Not only do we have a broad choice of foods (in fact, we're surrounded by food at almost every moment), but many of our processed foods have been vitamin- or mineral-fortified: milk has added vitamins A and D, and sometimes also zinc, iron and folic acid; fruit juices often have added calcium; and breads and cereals usually incorporate a panoply of added nutrients, including folic acid and various B vitamins. According to the Academy of Nutrition and Dietetics, the majority of Americans get enough of most nutrients without taking supplements.

Does this status change if you're following an intermittent fasting program? Not really, says Michael Mosley, MD, author of *The Fast Diet*. "On an intermittent method, which is not a deprivation regimen, your nutritional intake from a wide variety of food

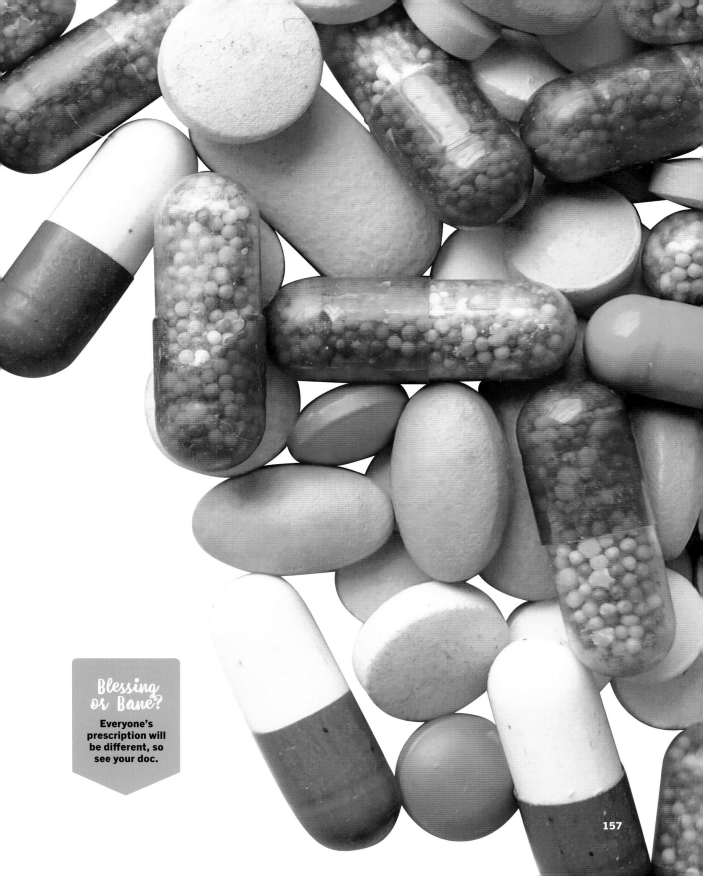

Blessing
or Bane?

**Everyone's prescription will be different, so see your doc.**

sources should remain relatively steady over time," Mosley says. You should, he adds, focus on taking in high-quality fresh foods, including healthy protein sources and plant foods, on both fasting days (if you are doing 5:2, which includes a small amount of calories while fasting) and feasting days. "They'll give you all the goodness you need without resorting to costly bottled multivitamins," he says.

There are two other things to take into account when considering supplements. One is that the entire $32 billion-a-year industry is essentially unregulated. Since the passage of the Dietary Supplement Health and Education Act of 1994, all dietary supplements have been presumed to be safe, because they're derived from natural substances. So unlike drug companies, supplement manufacturers don't have to run clinical trials, consult federal regulators or offer any proof that their products work—or even that they do no harm. No surprise that supplement makers have flooded the markets since then. Multiple studies have shown great variation in the quality of supplement products, with some containing very little of their purported ingredient.

The other consideration is that some supplements that were widely hailed—for instance, beta-carotene and vitamin E—have been shown in studies to actually be harmful in large doses. Why would this be? Many experts have speculated that while various nutrients have been proven to be beneficial when they occur naturally in foods,

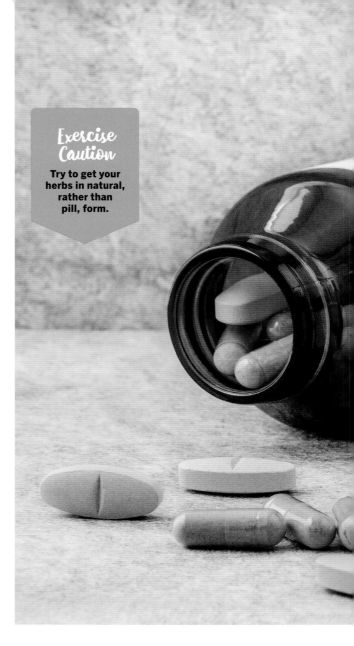

**Exercise Caution**

Try to get your herbs in natural, rather than pill, form.

✕

# ANNOYED BY CRAVINGS? CERTAIN MINERALS, AMINO ACIDS AND HERBS CAN HELP.

it doesn't necessarily follow that taking massive, concentrated doses of those nutrients in pill form is as good, or better—or even safe. "There might be synergistic effects among the various components in foods," says Carol Haggans, MS, RD, a scientific and health communications consultant for the National Institutes of Health (NIH). "You can't completely duplicate the food in pill form." Nutrition studies are often based on entire

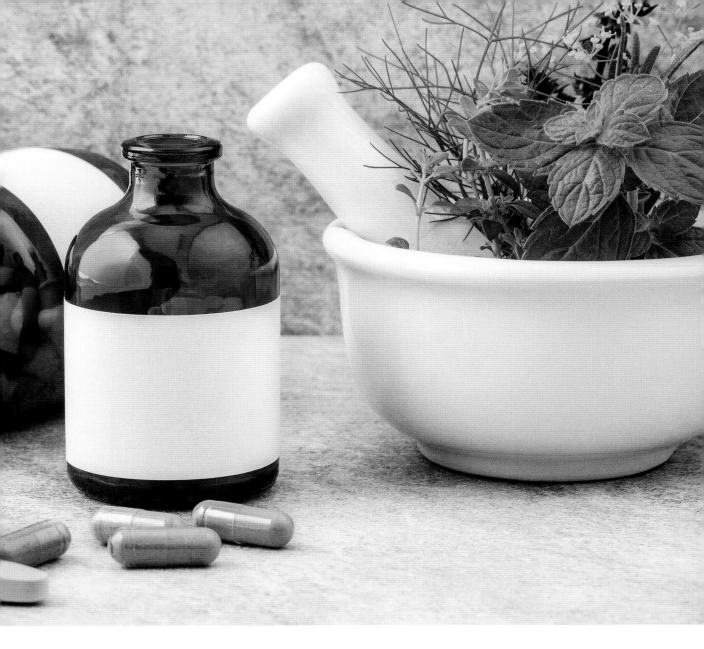

populations, but it's hard to know whether health benefits are coming from, say, the omega-3s in fish, or from other aspects of a fish-eating lifestyle.

In addition, supplements are bioactive and thus not always harmless. A study in the *New England Journal of Medicine* found that more than 23,000 emergency room visits per year are linked with negative effects from supplements, which may be worsened by fasting.

## If the Answer Is Yes

So you do want to take some supplements? No problem—but there are a few things you should know. First, time your vitamin-swallowing around whatever food you're taking in. "Taking vitamins on an empty stomach can frequently upset the GI tract," says gastroenterologist Christine Lee, MD. "Many people experience stomach pains, nausea and even diarrhea." Vitamins and supplements

**159**

can also aggravate any preexisting digestive conditions, like acid reflux, ulcers, gastritis or irritable bowel syndrome, Lee adds.

To be safe, take supplements during your eating times, whether it's a mini-meal on 5:2, or the eight-hour eating window on 16:8. If you're doing a longer fast, experts agree it's safer to refrain from pills when your stomach is entirely empty.

Some fasting experts, however, feel that certain natural supplements may help with both fat-burning and hunger. Julian Whitaker, MD, founder of the Whitaker Wellness Institute, recommends looking up these ingredients—although he also emphasizes that any of these are entirely optional:

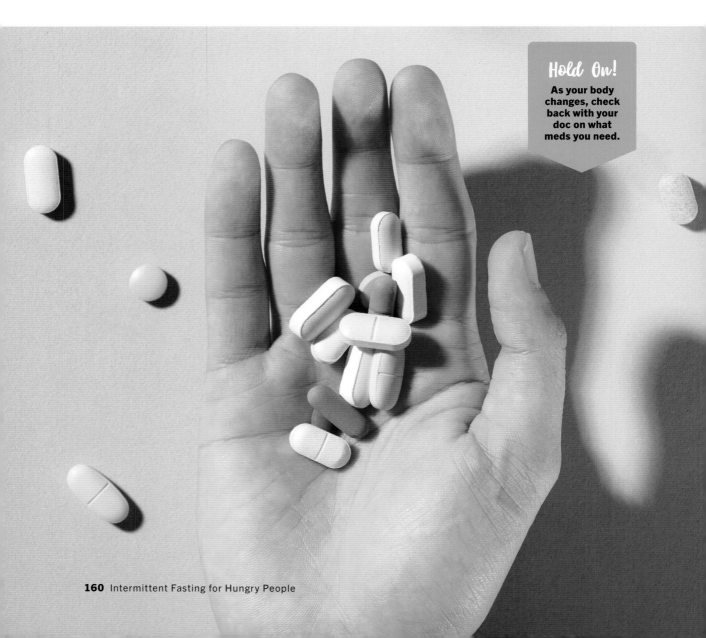

### Hold On!

**As your body changes, check back with your doc on what meds you need.**

### HYDROXYCITRIC ACID (HCA)

✳ An herbal extract from the rind of a fruit traditionally used in India, HCA may stimulate the activity of an enzyme that enables fat to be burned in the liver, and also boosts the production of ketones (which fuel the brain and reduce food cravings).

### CHROMIUM

✳ A trace mineral that enhances the activity of insulin and is involved in carbohydrate, fat and protein metabolism, chromium may help stabilize blood sugar and reduce hunger and cravings.

### 5-HYDROXYTRYPTOPHAN (5-HTP)

✳ A precursor to serotonin, the "happiness" neurotransmitter, this natural amino acid may help curb appetite and reduce carb cravings.

### SAFFRON

✳ An herbal extract that has been shown to increase serotonin levels and reduce stress eating.

## What About Medications?

If you are on any prescription meds, your first step is to visit your doctor, says Jason Fung, MD, co-founder of the Intensive Dietary Management Program. This is especially the case if your meds treat a condition that may be affected by IF, such as high blood pressure or diabetes. "Metformin, used for diabetes but also sometimes prescribed for other conditions, like polycystic ovary syndrome, may cause nausea or diarrhea if taken on an empty stomach," Fung says.

But the larger question is whether your prescription strength will need to be adjusted, he cautions. "Blood pressure can sometimes become low during a fast," says Fung. "If you take blood pressure medications, you may find that your blood pressure becomes too low, which can cause lightheadedness." Keep in close touch with your doctor about possibly changing your dosage, and monitor your BP with a home device.

The same cautions hold with diabetes medications. "Fasting reduces blood sugars," Fung explains. In general that's good, but

## Supplements to Consider

These four may supply a boost during fasting:

### MULTIVITAMINS

There's no harm in taking a good multi (just not on an empty stomach) to cover your bases, but "don't expect miracles," says Carol Haggans, MS, RD, of the NIH. "Most research shows that they don't reduce the risk of chronic diseases such as cancer or heart disease."

### VITAMIN D

Many people, especially those in less-sunny climates, come up short on this nutrient.

### CALCIUM

If you are lacking in calcium, your body will "steal" it from your bones. Combine it with vitamin D for the maximum benefits.

### FIBER

A natural source, like psyllium, can help with any digestive issues.

"if you're taking diabetic medications, especially insulin, your blood sugars may become extremely low, which can be life-threatening. Close monitoring of your blood sugars with your physician is mandatory," he cautions. If fasting is working for you, your meds may very well need to be reduced, Fung adds: "In the Intensive Dietary Management Program, we often reduce medications before starting a fast, in anticipation of lower blood sugars." The good news: If you're a Type 2 diabetic, and IF lowers your blood sugar, you may eventually be able to go off your medications.

If you're taking any other daily meds, the best fasting plan may be one that allows you at least one solid meal a day—like 16:8 or OMAD/Warrior. That will help protect against any stomach upset.

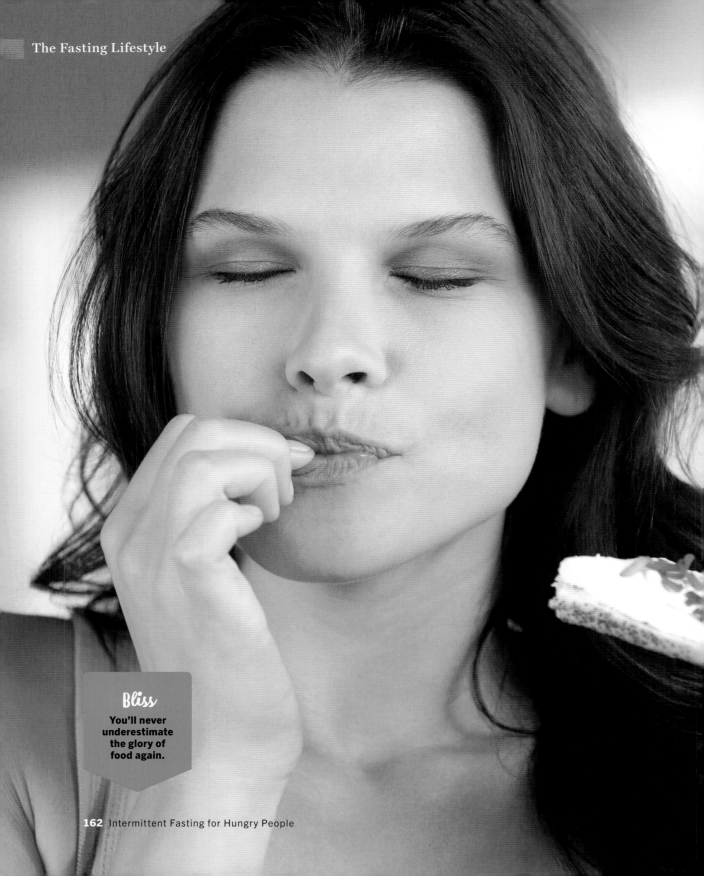

### Bliss

**You'll never underestimate the glory of food again.**

# THE GIFT OF
# EATING
## MINDFULLY

**Fasting will change the way you think of food—
in the best possible way.**

**WHO KNEW THAT** a dietary regimen focused on *not* eating could transform the way you experience eating itself? Intermittent fasting can do exactly that, in part by turning your attention away from the minutia of calories, the juggling of macronutrients and, especially, the judgments about food that come with traditional diets. Many experts feel that those judgments—this food is "sinful," that food is "right" or "good"—have damaged our relationship with what we eat and dulled our ability to distinguish true hunger from simple cravings. And by "outlawing" certain foods, we've endowed them with superpowers they shouldn't have. Fasting brings hunger back into the equation (the "when" of eating), while doing away with the strictures (the "what" of it). The result: considerably more pleasure, and potentially better health.

Here's how it works. First, when you graze your way through the day—from breakfast to snacks at the office to dinner, then cookies or popcorn—your body never gets the chance to become truly hungry. So your eating becomes driven by external events, like "It's time for lunch" or "Someone brought doughnuts to the conference room!" Then, when you layer on rules ("But I shouldn't eat the doughnuts!"), you diverge even further from any sense of what you really need to eat, says Tracy Brown, RD, who counsels clients in intuitive and what she calls "attuned" eating. "If you've been 'watching your food' in any way—and that includes 'trying to eat healthy'—you may have trouble distinguishing between physical hunger and 'symbolic hunger.'"

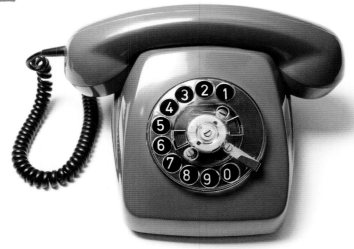

## PUT AWAY THE PHONE AND TURN OFF THE COMPUTER OR TV: NOW IS YOUR TIME TO FOCUS ON THE FLAVORS YOU'LL FIND IN EVERY BITE.

And as everyone knows, eating when you're not truly hungry just isn't that satisfying.

This confusion about hunger short-circuits our innate sensor that tells us when to eat and when to stop, says Alexis Conason, PsyD, a clinical psychologist in New York City, researcher at Mount Sinai Morningside hospital, and the founder of The Anti-Diet Plan. "Kids will naturally do this, before they become disconnected from their own bodies, which happens when they get old enough to absorb the conflicts our culture has about pleasure and food. My 4-year-old daughter will leave half a bowl of ice cream, which she loves, once she's full."

Fasting gets us back to that inborn ability to eat what we need. It also allows us to rediscover the pure joy of food—because nothing tastes better than that first meal after a fasting period. If you incorporate the tenets of mindful eating in conjunction with intermittent fasting, you'll approach food as the fulfilling, even spiritual, experience it can be. Because even as fasting has long had a spiritual element, so too does feeding our souls along with our bodies. Here's how to do that with IF.

### Mindful Eating While Fasting

If you're following an alternate-day or 5:2 plan, you will have days when you consume only about 500 to 600 calories, so make them count, advises

Los Angeles–based nutritionist Cynthia Sass, MPH, RD. "On fasting days, make a conscious effort to slow your eating pace," says Sass. "Take small bites, and remove mealtime distractions like the TV or phone. Both actions have been shown to boost satiety." If you're on time-restricted feeding, try to experience the drinks you're taking in, whether tea or bone broth, with the same pleasure and appreciation.

### Mindful Eating After Fasting

First, slow down! You'll be truly hungry, and it can be tempting to wolf your food, which won't be pleasurable. "Eat a little bit, then pause to allow your blood sugar to come back up, so you can think clearly and make mindful decisions," says Michelle May, PhD, author of the book series *Eat What You Love, Love What You Eat*. Then apply the actions of mindful eating: Examine your food visually, smelling it, feeling it, slowly biting into it, sensing its flavor and texture. Try to experience it as if you've never encountered it before. In one study, some participants were assigned the task of eating a raisin mindfully, while others (the control group) simply ate raisins. Then everyone was offered an array of food. The mindful group reported significantly higher levels of enjoyment of the later food samples, just from one try at mindful eating. Mission accomplished!

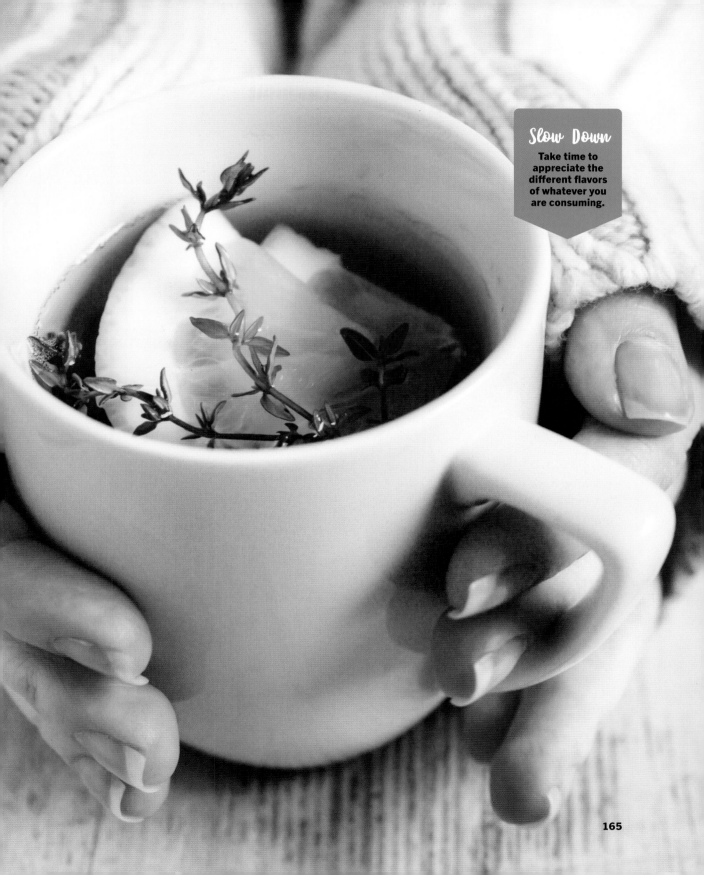

**Slow Down**
Take time to
appreciate the
different flavors
of whatever you
are consuming.

165

# THE
# ULTIMATE
## CHALLENGE

**How do you fast when your whole life revolves around food? These high-profile chefs—all of whom lost weight on IF—have some answers.**

## SCOTT CONANT

**FAT AND HAPPY**—that's my motto," Scott Conant told an audience of foodies as he added an obscene amount of cream and butter to an Italian dish called gnudi during a cooking demo at the USA Today Wine & Food Experience in Chicago one November. It may be his motto, but it's not one he lives by anymore. The chef, restaurant owner and cookbook author, who appears regularly on *Chopped* and *Top Chef*, lost 30 pounds by giving up alcohol and wheat while following an intermittent fasting plan.

Wheat was first to go. What might have been difficult for the average carb-lover seems downright impossible for an Italian chef. "It's ironic because I am a chef who is known for cooking pasta," Conant told *People* magazine. "But I stopped eating wheat on a daily basis. Now I just pretty much do it for work."

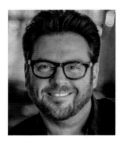

Conant was soon rewarded with a 12-pound weight loss after cutting out wheat for just 10 days. The additional 18 pounds came off only after he started a regimen of both IF and working out.

His program: He fasts for 17 out of 24 hours, and usually only eats from noon to 7 p.m. Breakfast is coffee or hot water with lemon; for lunch it's chicken or salmon with salad; dinner is a protein with vegetables. "I've fallen off a couple times," he told *People*. "I travel a lot. I always seem to be on the road, so I think it is easy to fall back into old habits."

The trick, he said, is to cut yourself some slack and get back on track. "I'm a big believer in moderation and not killing myself," said Conant. "I do not overindulge. But I also do not beat myself up if I have a bowl of pasta. The next day is a new day."

He also reports his clothes seem to fit better, and that colleagues have complimented his now-slimmer physique.

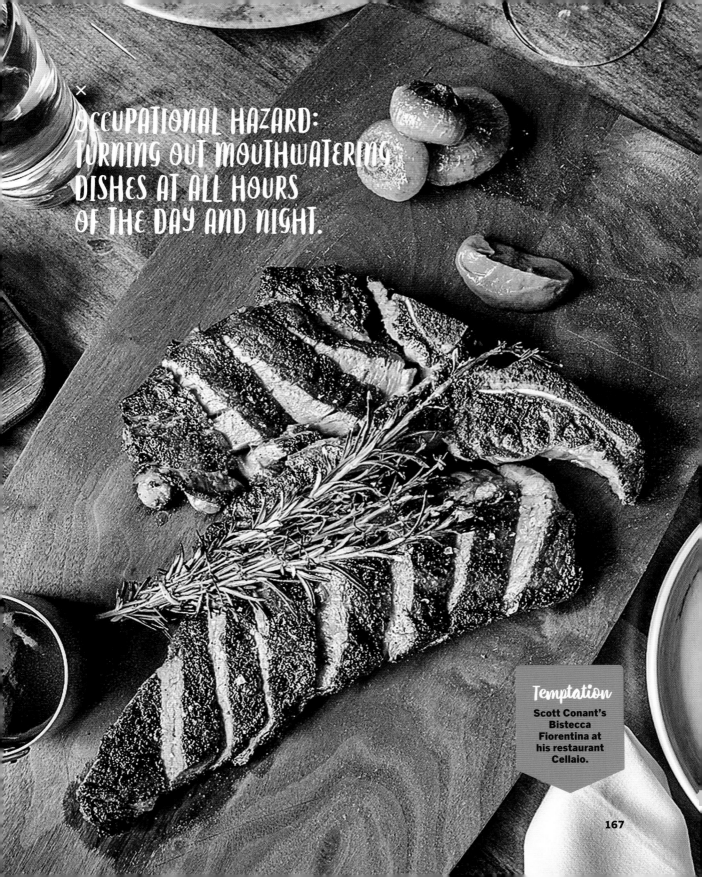

OCCUPATIONAL HAZARD: TURNING OUT MOUTHWATERING DISHES AT ALL HOURS OF THE DAY AND NIGHT.

## Temptation

Scott Conant's Bistecca Fiorentina at his restaurant Cellaio.

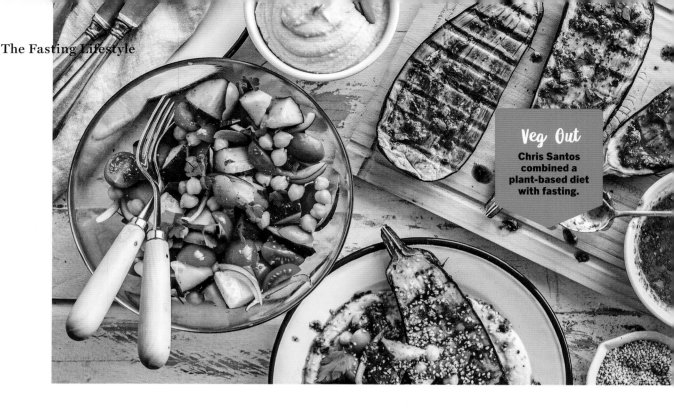

**Veg Out**
Chris Santos combined a plant-based diet with fasting.

# CHRIS SANTOS

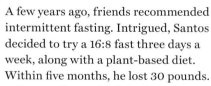

**IF YOU COUNT** yourself among the Food Network faithful—or, more specifically, a faithful fan of *Chopped*—you may have wondered over the years: Is it just me, or does Chris Santos seem to be slowly packing on the pounds? The quick answers: No, it wasn't just you. And yes, Santos was putting on weight. "Over the course of 10 years, I gained 50 pounds, which is a ton of weight," the chef and *Chopped* judge told *People* magazine. "If you think about it, it's 5 pounds a year, which is less than half a pound a month. It just kind of gradually went on and on and on."

That's what happens when you're running upscale restaurants with multiple locations (like Beauty & Essex, which expanded from New York City to Las Vegas and Los Angeles). Santos' long hours often had him getting home late at night and ordering a takeout dinner of cheesesteak, pizza or a cheeseburger. "If GrubHub had a category called 'unhealthy,' that would be the one I would be clicking on every time," he said.

A few years ago, friends recommended intermittent fasting. Intrigued, Santos decided to try a 16:8 fast three days a week, along with a plant-based diet. Within five months, he lost 30 pounds.

Santos also cut back on his beer intake, and instead indulges in vodka and soda or whiskey with water. He has taken up running. And he allows himself a "cheat day." To keep it under control, he and his girlfriend have a deal. "She just knows what it means when I say, 'Take this,'" Santos said. "She knows that it means get it away, or I'll keep eating it if it sits in front of me."

✕

A RESTAURANT CRITIC DESCRIBED SANTOS' FOOD AS "SEXY...AND OUTRAGEOUSLY FLAVORFUL."

# MiKE DeCAMP

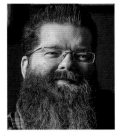

**WHEN YOU'RE THE** culinary director at a company that owns five restaurants, you get to do things like order pancakes or a porterhouse on a whim, snack on lamb sliders no matter the hour, or ask one of your chefs to whip up, well, you name it. But then one day you wake up and realize that the coolest thing about your job is also the thing that's sabotaging your health.

That's pretty much what happened to Mike DeCamp, who works for Jester Concepts, the hospitality company behind some of Minneapolis and St. Paul, Minnesota's most popular restaurants, including P.S. Steak.

The question was: How would DeCamp lose the weight? Following a strict diet would be tricky, given his work schedule. He needed an eating plan that didn't restrict certain foods or prohibit the kind of grazing that's all in a day's work.

That's what appealed to him about intermittent fasting: He could fast for 16 hours a day and then eat during work hours, between 5 p.m. and 1 a.m., a window that allows him to sample dishes and specials throughout the evening, and then eat dinner around 11 p.m. when he gets home. That may not be the schedule most people follow on 16:8, but for DeCamp it was magic.

After a month, he'd dropped several pants sizes. But something else happened that he hadn't necessarily expected. As DeCamp told *Cooking Light* magazine, his "mental fogginess" lifted and his improved energy levels inspired him to take up cycling again and eat fewer inflammatory foods.

"[Intermittent fasting] has shown me that if I have the willpower to maintain a style of eating, then I can have the willpower to eat better, too," DeCamp said. "It has really changed my attitude toward food." Now 55 pounds lighter, he tries to "eat as many plant-based items that I can and consume a smaller amount of meat."

His advice for anyone beginning an intermittent fasting plan? "Start by pushing yourself in uncomfortable ways, little by little, until you feel like you can do more," said DeCamp. "That might mean eating better at just one meal a day to start, and gradually making all meals more healthy. Try to make it as enjoyable as you can, so that it becomes a lifestyle instead of just a diet."

✕

## PROOF OF INTERMITTENT FASTING'S FLEXIBILITY: DECAMP DOESN'T OPEN HIS EATING WINDOW UNTIL 5 P.M.

## Green Day

**Mike DeCamp has also cut down drastically on meat in favor of plants.**

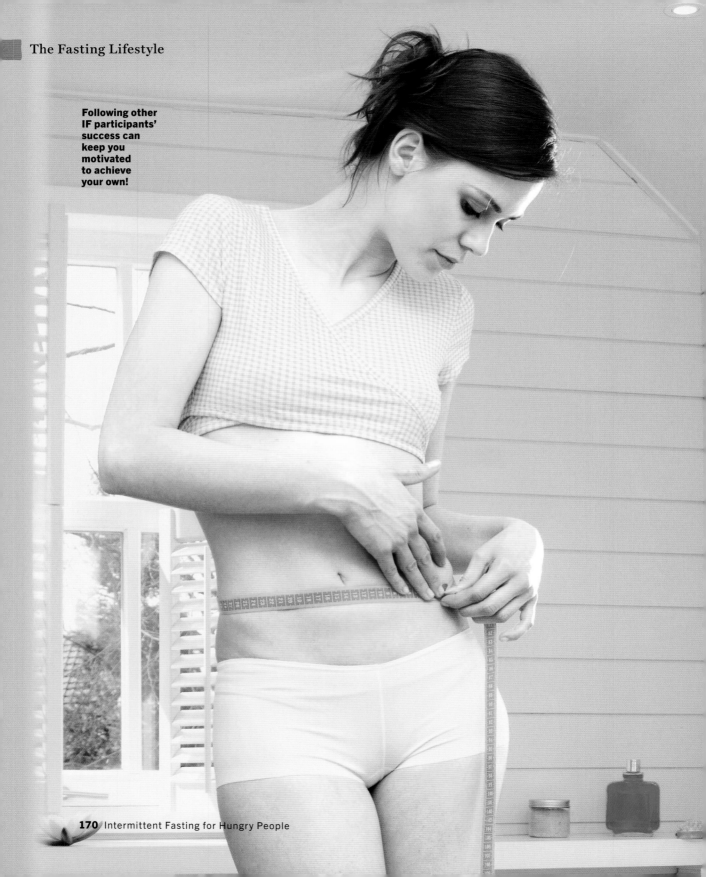

**Following other IF participants' success can keep you motivated to achieve your own!**

# REAL-LIFE
# SUCCESS
## STORIES

**Seeking inspiration? Thousands of people have been helped by intermittent fasting. Here's how three of them lost weight and gained health and energy through IF.**

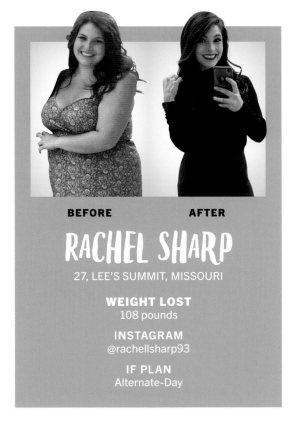

**BEFORE**     **AFTER**

## RACHEL SHARP
27, LEE'S SUMMIT, MISSOURI

**WEIGHT LOST**
108 pounds

**INSTAGRAM**
@rachellsharp93

**IF PLAN**
Alternate-Day

**HER STORY** "I had been overweight since I was a little girl, and was badly bullied for it all through school," says Sharp, who describes herself back then as shy and lacking in confidence and self-esteem—largely because of her weight. After high school, she tried a litany of weight-loss methods, none of which had an effect. Finally, two years ago, she went on a hike with a new boyfriend (now her husband) and could barely keep up. "My feet hurt, my knees ached, I was struggling to breathe. I was so ashamed of myself. Something had to change."

That "something" turned out to be IF, and it changed everything. Her then-boyfriend was doing the 16:8 method for health reasons, but Sharp was skeptical at first. Then she saw an article by a woman who followed an alternate-day IF method (ADF), and Sharp jumped on the bandwagon. "I decided to start my own method of ADF, going every other day, or 36 to 40 hours, without eating, while also counting calories." During her first week, Sharp allowed herself up to 500 calories on fasting days to "wean" herself into going 40 hours without food. "I didn't really change much of what I was eating, beyond

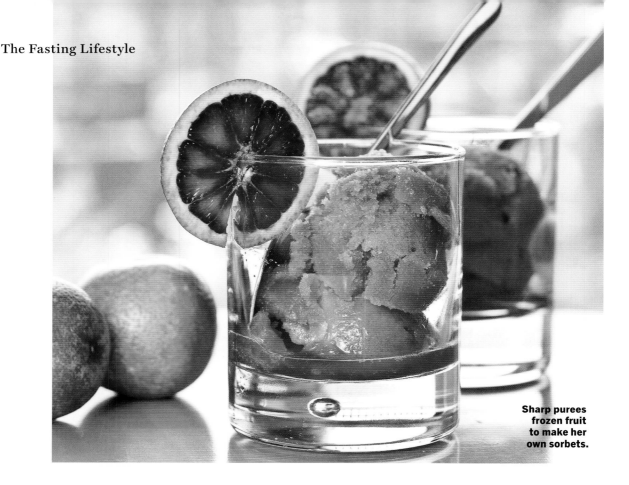

**Sharp purees frozen fruit to make her own sorbets.**

watching the calories I was taking in. By the second week, I could go the whole fasting day without taking in any calories at all. IF was a lot easier than I thought it would be!"

Only after she got used to her new eating schedule did Sharp concentrate on swapping out less nutritious meals for healthier ones. "I changed little things, like going from 2% milk to almond milk," she says. On a typical nonfasting day, she might eat oatmeal with fruit for breakfast, cauliflower rice with shrimp or beef for lunch, and baked chicken with vegetables for dinner. Dessert might be frozen fruit blended in a food processor ("Healthy sorbet!").

"After one month of ADF I lost 16 pounds," she says. "I was elated!" Seven months later—down 62 pounds—Sharp started working out for the first time. "I went from hardly being able to jog for two minutes, to running for 20 to 28 minutes without

stopping," she says. After a year of ADF, and down 98 pounds, she added in weightlifting. Now she runs on fasting days and lifts on eating days: "This is the perfect balance for me."

**HER ADVICE** "Going without eating can sometimes be difficult, and you have to listen to your body. If it's really nagging at you, just eat—you can have up to 500 calories without disrupting your fasting day. I've also found that if I stay busy on my fasting days, I'm much more likely to stick with it. Whenever I feel discouraged or unmotivated, I remember why I started. My weight-loss experience has revealed the true me, and I don't ever want to go back to the girl I used to be. I wish I knew I had this type of willpower and strength in me all along, because I've overcome so many obstacles since starting that I never thought I would achieve."

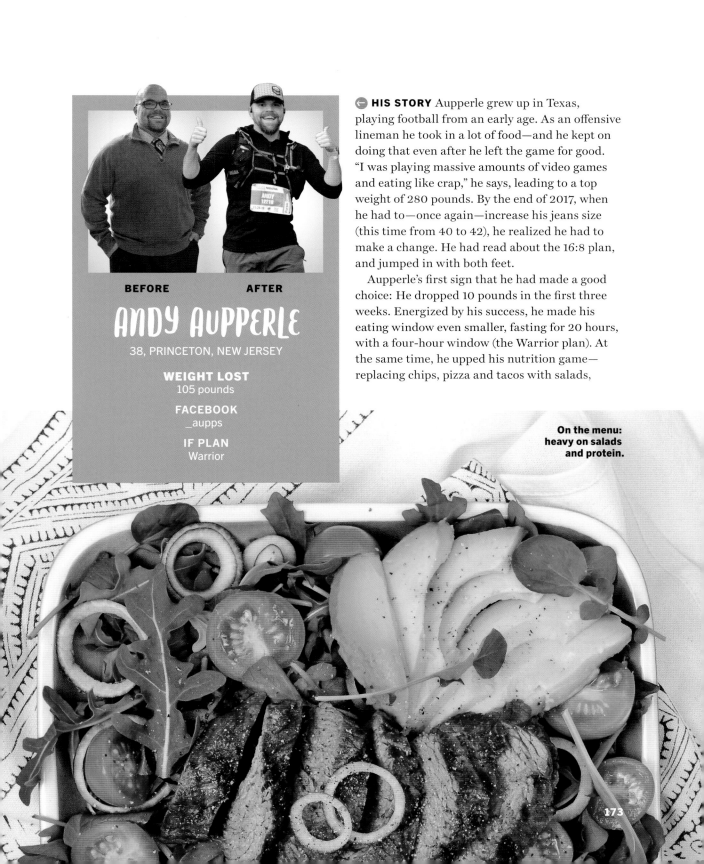

**BEFORE** **AFTER**

# ANDY AUPPERLE

38, PRINCETON, NEW JERSEY

**WEIGHT LOST**
105 pounds

**FACEBOOK**
_aupps

**IF PLAN**
Warrior

**HIS STORY** Aupperle grew up in Texas, playing football from an early age. As an offensive lineman he took in a lot of food—and he kept on doing that even after he left the game for good. "I was playing massive amounts of video games and eating like crap," he says, leading to a top weight of 280 pounds. By the end of 2017, when he had to—once again—increase his jeans size (this time from 40 to 42), he realized he had to make a change. He had read about the 16:8 plan, and jumped in with both feet.

Aupperle's first sign that he had made a good choice: He dropped 10 pounds in the first three weeks. Energized by his success, he made his eating window even smaller, fasting for 20 hours, with a four-hour window (the Warrior plan). At the same time, he upped his nutrition game— replacing chips, pizza and tacos with salads,

**On the menu: heavy on salads and protein.**

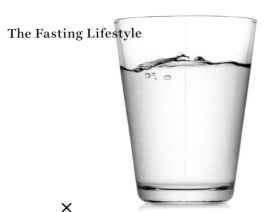

## "HUNGER PAINS ARE JUST YOUR MIND HAVING A TANTRUM. DRINK SOME WATER; THEY'LL PASS," SAYS AUPPERLE.

vegetables and chicken—and took up running. It was tough at first, Aupperle says. "I was slow and got winded so easily. It wasn't pretty at all, but I did like being outside, so I kept doing it." He set small goals, like going two minutes without stopping, then kept lengthening the intervals. Eventually he was running 5Ks, and adding in yoga and body-weight workouts.

All of that activity put him on a steady path of losing about 15 pounds a month. By November of that year, 11 months after starting with IF, he had hit his goal weight of 175 pounds. At that point, he says, some of his friends hardly recognized him: "Nobody had seen me skinny before." Aupperle now feels good in his skin, as well as being far more energetic, leading him to train for, and complete, his first marathon in November 2019. "I'm super proud of that," he says.

**HIS ADVICE** To anyone else following an IF plan and trying to get in shape, he says, "It's going to take time for it to come off—after all, it took 35 years to put on all that weight—but the results will come."

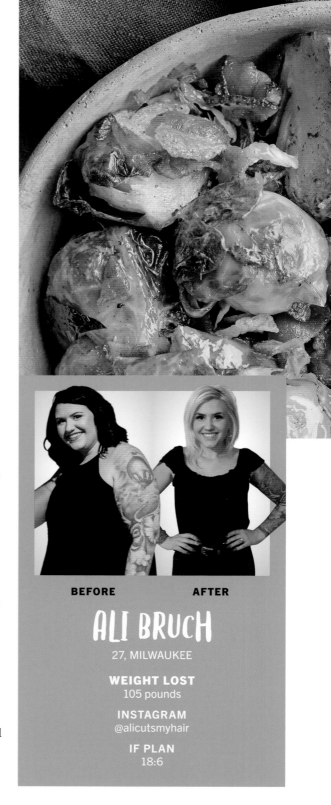

**BEFORE**      **AFTER**

## ALI BRUCH

27, MILWAUKEE

**WEIGHT LOST**
105 pounds

**INSTAGRAM**
@alicutsmyhair

**IF PLAN**
18:6

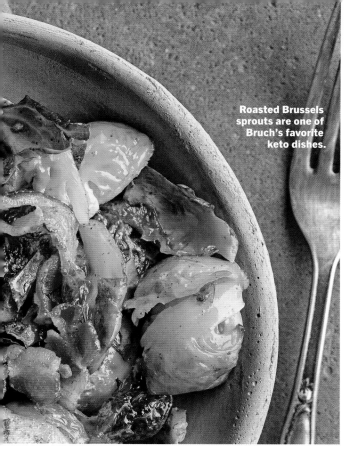

**Roasted Brussels sprouts are one of Bruch's favorite keto dishes.**

🔙 **HER STORY** Bruch had been overweight her entire life—"well, morbidly obese, if I'm being honest," she admits. At her heaviest she reached 270 pounds, and it affected her life in profound ways. Working on her feet all day as a hairstylist was physically painful, and she would come home with swollen ankles. Running around with her young daughter became impossible.

"I would hide whenever someone took pictures," Bruch says. "I was afraid they'd get posted online, and people would know how big I really was." Looking back, she considers herself a binge eater—"When I started eating, I couldn't stop"— sometimes taking in up to 8,000 calories a day. "It makes me sad to think of how I treated my body."

Bruch received a wake-up call in 2016, when she was shopping for a wedding dress. "The saleswoman made it very clear to me that the 'normal-sized' dresses wouldn't fit me—I had to look at the plus-size options." Humiliated, Bruch left the shop. Soon after, she saw an Instagram post about weight loss with the keto diet, and it "lit a fire inside me," says Bruch. Even though it was one day before Halloween, the biggest sugar-high holiday of the year, she jumped on the keto train. Soon she added IF, eventually cutting her eating window down to six hours (18:6 time-restricted feeding). "I fast from 6 in the evening until noon the next day, and break my fast with lunch," Bruch says.

The combination of keto and IF was, finally, a livable weight-loss method for Bruch—who has lost more than 100 pounds. "Calorie-counting and Weight Watchers are both great—but for me, they gave me too much flexibility." Cutting out most carbs and eating over six hours, on the other hand, offers Bruch just the right amount of structure. On a typical day she consumes black coffee and water till noon, then breaks the fast with salads containing meat (taco salad is a favorite) or homemade egg salad in a lettuce "wrap." Dinner might be a burger with no bun, and Brussels sprouts with bacon, followed by a piece of Lily's chocolate.

**HER ADVICE** "Set small goals. It feels a lot better to often reach small goals than to feel like you have one giant overall goal still out of reach. So I would set a [weight-loss] goal of just 2 to 3 pounds, and if that takes a week or a month, that's OK—I still have my large goal in mind. Then I set a new small goal. I take one day at a time."

✕

# "I REMIND MYSELF ON HARD DAYS TO 'JUST GET THROUGH TODAY.' STUFF HAPPENS—DON'T GIVE UP," SAYS BRUCH.

# THE NEW DIET OF THE STARS

The benefits of intermittent fasting have caught on with athletes, actors, reality stars and others who are in the public eye. Check out why they took the plunge.

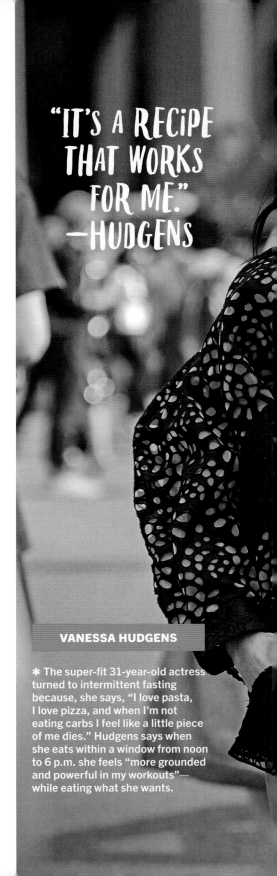

"IT'S A RECIPE THAT WORKS FOR ME." —HUDGENS

**VANESSA HUDGENS**

✱ The super-fit 31-year-old actress turned to intermittent fasting because, she says, "I love pasta, I love pizza, and when I'm not eating carbs I feel like a little piece of me dies." Hudgens says when she eats within a window from noon to 6 p.m. she feels "more grounded and powerful in my workouts"— while eating what she wants.

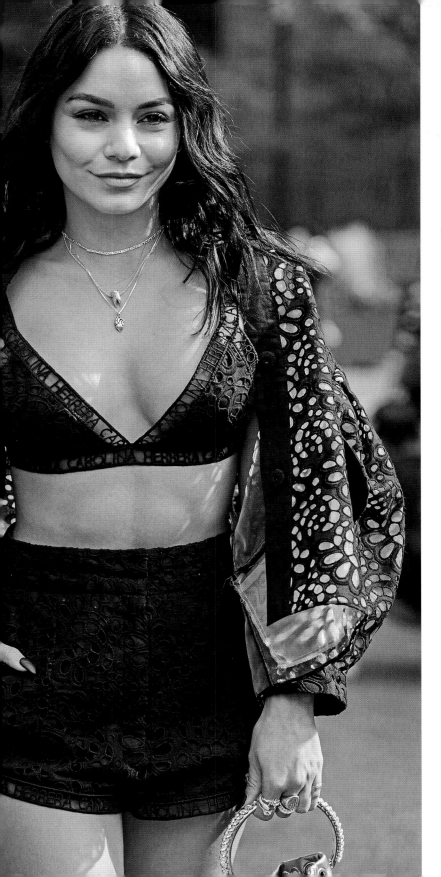

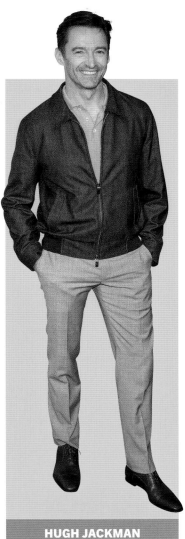

**HUGH JACKMAN**

✳ The Australian actor has played everything from a wolverine to a song-and-dance man, and at 51, his roles show him maintaining his cut and lean physique. He says he stays that way partly due to 16:8 IF, which Dwayne "The Rock" Johnson introduced to him. "Every day I eat for eight hours and I fast for 16," Jackman says. "From 10 in the morning till 6, I eat way too much, and then nothing after that. It's very unsocial! But I've found that 70 percent of how you look is your diet, as opposed to workouts and weightlifting."

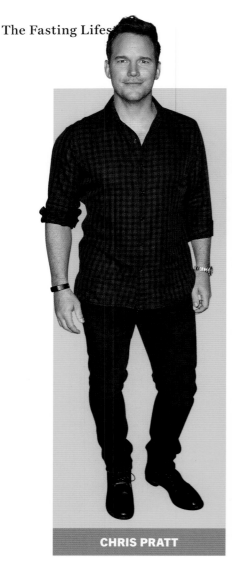

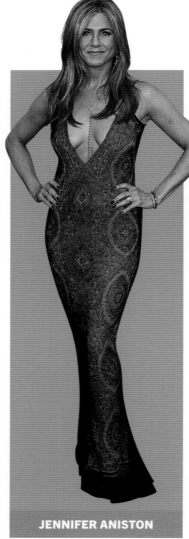

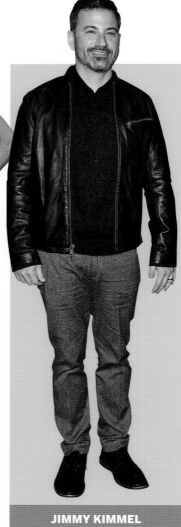

**CHRIS PRATT**

**JENNIFER ANISTON**

**JIMMY KIMMEL**

✳ "I'm doing this intermittent fasting thing," the *Jurassic World* star wrote on Instagram in 2018. "I get my cardio in during the morning, and then I finally get my coffee with oat milk." The 41-year-old gives the 16:8 plan a thumbs-up, writing, "Look it up, check it out, it's actually kinda cool. It works pretty well, and I've lost a little weight so far."

"I DON'T EAT TILL NOON."—PRATT

✳ The 51-year-old actress has maintained her figure since her *Friends* days, and her latest weapon is IF. "I do intermittent fasting, so no food in the morning," Aniston has said. "I noticed a big difference in going without solid food for 16 hours." She has tweaked the 16:8 plan in one way: She likes to start her day with a celery juice around 9 a.m., while fasting purists hold off on everything but water, tea and coffee. Considering that one cup of celery juice has all of 40 calories, though, it may not be a deal-breaker.

✳ The 52-year-old comedian and talk-show host has test-driven two different forms of IF, 16:8 and 5:2. First he ate within a window, consuming two protein shakes and then a small dinner each day. The result: a 25-pound loss. Then he moved to a plan where, as he puts it, "On Monday and Thursday, I eat fewer than 500 calories a day, then I eat like a pig for the other five days. You 'surprise' the body, keep it guessing. It sounds hard, but you get used to it and learn you can get through it. It's made me appreciate the food that I do eat."

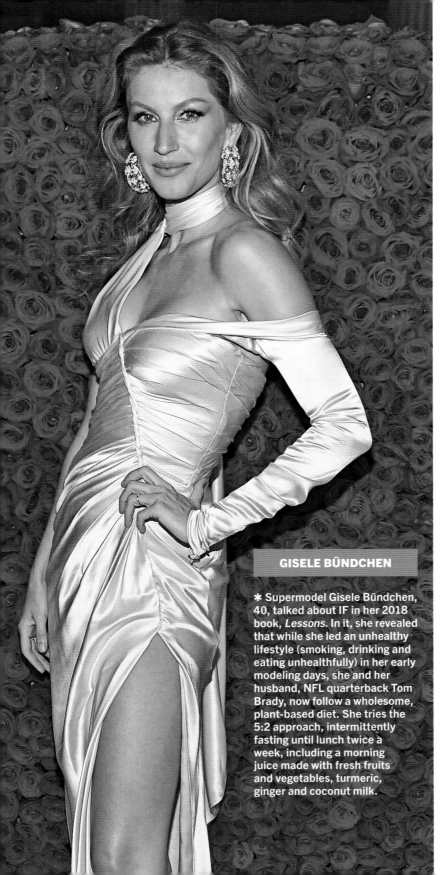

## GISELE BÜNDCHEN

✻ Supermodel Gisele Bündchen, 40, talked about IF in her 2018 book, *Lessons*. In it, she revealed that while she led an unhealthy lifestyle (smoking, drinking and eating unhealthfully) in her early modeling days, she and her husband, NFL quarterback Tom Brady, now follow a wholesome, plant-based diet. She tries the 5:2 approach, intermittently fasting until lunch twice a week, including a morning juice made with fresh fruits and vegetables, turmeric, ginger and coconut milk.

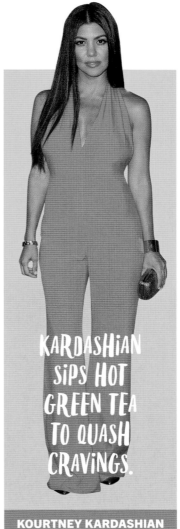

KARDASHIAN SIPS HOT GREEN TEA TO QUASH CRAVINGS.

## KOURTNEY KARDASHIAN

✻ This member of the Kardashian clan is known for trying all kinds of regimens, but she raves about fasting for 14 to 16 hours a day. "I don't eat past 7 p.m., and then I eat breakfast the next day after my morning workout, which is at 10:30 or 11," explains Kardashian, who is 41. She often breaks her fast with a collagen-protein drink containing 20 grams of collagen and 18 grams of protein, mixed with water. The best part about the eating "window," she says, is that she can eat plenty of food, but it reins in her late-night snacking.

179

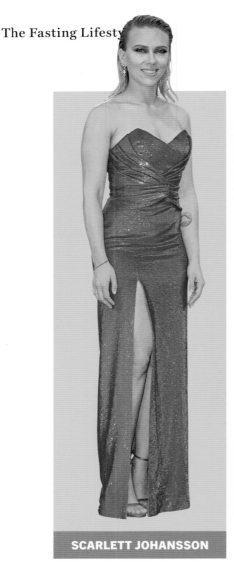

**SCARLETT JOHANSSON**

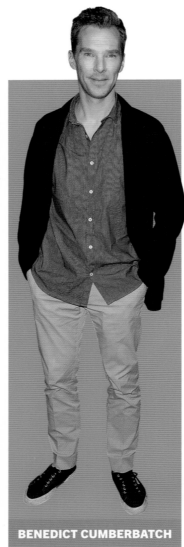

**BENEDICT CUMBERBATCH**

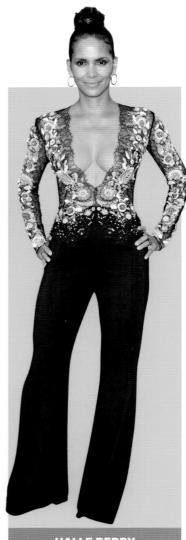

**HALLE BERRY**

✳ The Oscar-nominated actress, 35, wowed fans as Black Widow in *Avengers: Endgame* and is set to draw more buzz in the stand-alone movie about the deadly assassin. To prepare for the physically vigorous role, Johansson followed a demanding training regimen, which included a minimum of 12 hours of fasting every day. "That was a general guideline," her trainer Eric Johnson told *Harper's Bazaar* of her routine. "At moments we pushed beyond that to 14 to 15 hours depending on the filming schedule."

✳ When the 44-year-old British star had to transition from his buff superhero role in *Doctor Strange* to the lanky Sherlock Holmes, he turned to IF, eating very-low-calorie for two days a week. "I'm on the 5:2 plan," he told *The Times* of London. "You have to, for Sherlock."

**CUMBERBATCH GOES VERY LOW CAL FOR TWO DAYS.**

✳ The actress, 54, combines two hot plans: IF and keto. "I normally eat two meals a day," Berry wrote on Instagram. "I skip breakfast and sort of fast and do my green drink or my bullet coffee." She credits the coconut oil in her coffee with fueling her body and brain, and then breaks her fast with something like an egg-white omelet with red peppers and onions. Some people question whether bulletproof coffee is true IF, but others contend the pure fat simply adds to the production of ketones.

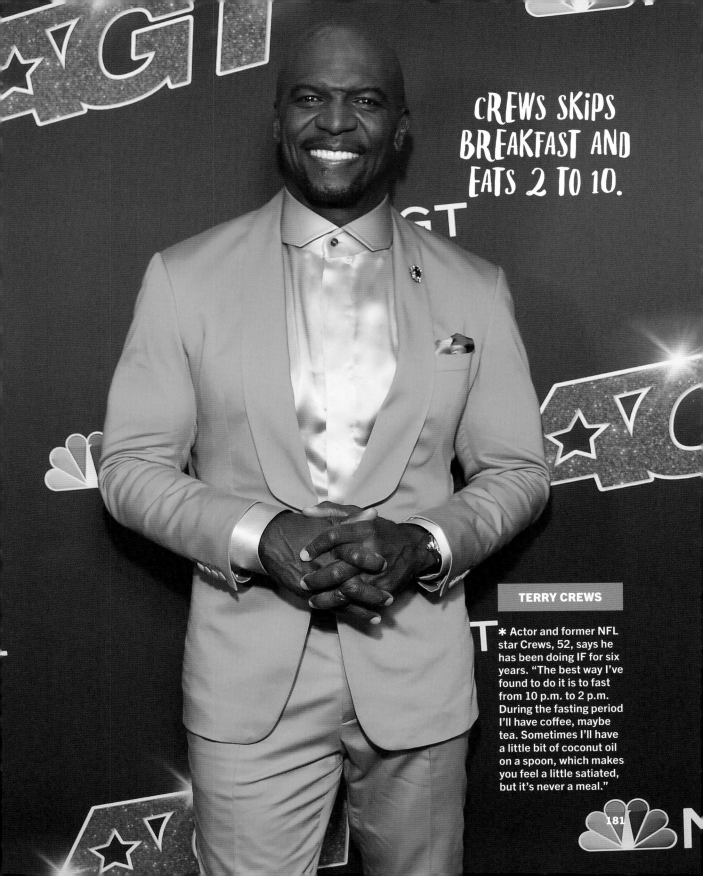

CREWS SKIPS
BREAKFAST AND
EATS 2 TO 10.

**TERRY CREWS**

✱ Actor and former NFL
star Crews, 52, says he
has been doing IF for six
years. "The best way I've
found to do it is to fast
from 10 p.m. to 2 p.m.
During the fasting period
I'll have coffee, maybe
tea. Sometimes I'll have
a little bit of coconut oil
on a spoon, which makes
you feel a little satiated,
but it's never a meal."

# YOUR INTERMITTENT FASTING
# WORKBOOK

Now that you know all that IF can do for you, it's time to
get into action! But before you do, take a few moments
to consider your motivation and your ultimate goals.

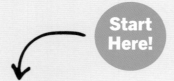 

**What made you decide to
give intermittent fasting a try?**

_____
_____
_____
_____
_____
_____
_____

**What are you hoping to get out
of doing an intermittent fasting
plan? What goals would you like
to reach?**

_____
_____
_____
_____
_____

**Why are these goals so
important to you?**

_____
_____
_____
_____
_____
_____

**Is your current lifestyle
in line with your goals?**

_____
_____
_____
_____
_____
_____
_____

**What worries do you have
about trying intermittent fasting?**

_____
_____
_____
_____
_____
_____
_____

**What would make you feel like
you've succeeded in following
an intermittent fasting plan?**

_____
_____
_____
_____
_____
_____

# WHAT DOES REACHING YOUR GOAL LOOK LIKE?

**Fill the spaces here with words, a collage or sketches of what your goal looks like in your mind.**

# WHAT INSPIRES YOU TO LIVE YOUR HEALTHIEST LIFE?

**Use the spaces here to think about who or what makes you want to look and feel your best.**

**What lifestyle changes would you like to make to help you reach your goals?**

_____
_____
_____
_____

**What makes you happy?**

_____
_____
_____
_____
_____

**What are some stumbling blocks you've had to deal with in the past when you've tried to make a change in your diet—and how can you overcome them now?**

_____
_____
_____
_____
_____
_____

**List three progress goals you would like to put in place to help you make these lifestyle changes.**

_____
_____
_____
_____

**Describe what feeling good is to you.**

_____
_____
_____
_____
_____

**What makes you excited about trying intermittent fasting?**

_____
_____
_____

**List five tools you have, or would like to have, in your personal toolbox to help keep worries, guilt, stress and bad feelings about dieting or yourself at bay.**

1 _____

2 _____

3 _____

4 _____

5 _____

**If you listed something you don't currently have in your life-skills toolbox (like meditation), can you think of some ways to incorporate this skill into your life?**

_____
_____
_____
_____
_____

# WHAT DOES A PERFECTLY HEALTHY DAY LOOK LIKE?

**Write out what you would consider to be your ideal day—then make it happen!**

# Index

# Index

# Credits

**COVER** Clockwise from main: Olga Miltsova/Shutterstock; Claudia Totir/Getty; Baibaz/ Getty; Pranom Panyacharoen/Shutterstock; Ken Carlson/Waterbury Publications; Nataly Studio/Shutterstock; Amenic181/Getty; Magone/Getty; Rustle/Shutterstock (background); Mama_mia/Shutterstock (spine) **INSIDE FRONT COVER** EllyGri/Shutterstock **2-3** Ella Olsson/@ellaolsson/Unsplash **4-5** Clockwise from bottom left: Chris Clor/Getty; Apichart Sripa/Shutterstock; Nadine Greefe/Stocksy; Yagi Studio/Getty; Enviromantic/Getty; Towfiqu Photography/Getty **6-7** Povpzniuk/Getty **8-9** Gilaxia/Getty **10-11** Elena Eryomenko/Shutterstock **12-13** JGI/Jamie Grill/Getty **14-15** Brett Stevens/Getty **16-17** Henrik5000/Getty **18-19** From left: SolStock/Getty; LdF/Getty **20-21** BlackJack3D/Getty **22-23** From left: Westend61/Getty; Andrew Brookes/Getty **24-25** From left: David Malan/Getty; Cavan Images/Getty **26-27** Apichart Sripa/Shutterstock **28-29** Aleksandra Voinova/Shutterstock **30-31** Westend61/Getty **32-33** PeopleImages/Getty **34-35** Plume Creative/Getty **36-37** JGI/Jamie Grill/Getty **38-39** Peter Dazeley/Getty **40-41** Vkillikov/Shutterstock **42-43** From left: Besedin/Shutterstock; Dimitrios/Shutterstock; Rawpixel.com/Shutterstock; Zvonimir Atletic/Shutterstock **44-45** Westend61/Getty **46-47** From left: Mama_mia/Shutterstock; Natasa Mandic/Stocksy **48-49** EllyGri/Shutterstock **50-51** Peopleimages/Getty **52-53** Westend61/Getty **54-55** Romolo Tavani/Getty **56-57** Zarzamora/Shutterstock **58-59** Satyrenko/Getty **60-61** Istetiana/Getty **62-63** From left: BonninStudio/Stocksy; LauriPatterson/Getty **64-65** Westend61/Getty **66** GMVozd/Getty **67** From left to right, Row 1: LoveTheWind/Getty; Issaurinko/Getty; StockPhotosArt/Shutterstock; Jultud/Getty; Valentyn Volkov/Shutterstock; Row 2: Baibaz/Getty; Assalve/Getty; Etorres69/Getty; Vovashevchuk/Getty; Tanya Sid/ Shutterstock; Row 3: Baibaz/Shutterstock; Alasdair James/Getty; Etienne Voss/Getty; Yeti Studio/Shutterstock; Francesco Perre/EyeEm/Getty; Row 4: Juanmonino/Getty; Creativ Studio Heinemann/Red Chopsticks Images/Getty; Ma-k/Getty; DebbiSmirnoff/ Getty; Xxmmxx/Getty **68-69** Mint Images/Getty **70-71** Rouzes/Getty **72-73** 10'000 Hours/Getty **74-75** Oleksandra Naumenko/Shutterstock **76-77** Enviromantic/Getty **78-79** JuliaK/Getty **80-81** Fotogal/Getty **82-83** Shapecharge/Getty **84-85** Elena Danileiko/Getty **86-87** Larissa Veronesi/Getty **88-89** From left: Yulkapopkova/Getty; Davies and Starr/Getty **90-91** Nadine Greefe/Stocksy **92-93** Vladislav Nosick/500px/Getty **94-95** Pixel Stories/Stocksy **96-97** Studio Firma/Stocksy **98-99** Westend61/Getty **100-101** From left: IriGri/Shutterstock; Hong Vo/Getty **102-103** From left: Anton Starikov/Shutterstock; Julija Dmitrijeva/Shutterstock **104-105** Sveta_Zarzamora/Getty **106-107** Clockwise from left: Thorsten Kraska/Getty; Ruta Lipskija/EyeEm/Getty; Sean De Burca/Getty **108-109** From left: Chris Clor/Getty; Roy Morsch/Getty **110-111** From left: Tracey Kusiewicz/Foodie Photography/Getty; Jenny Dettrick/Getty **112-113** Brian Hagiwara/Getty **114-115** From left: Yagi Studio/Getty; Jenifoto/Getty **116-117** Clockwise from left: Tijana Drndarski/@izgubljenausvemiru/Unsplash; Madeleine_Steinbach/Getty; Achim Sass/Getty **118-119** PeopleImages/Getty **120-121** Vasily Pindyurin/Getty **122-123** From left: Kamon Saejueng/EyeEm/Getty;Daxiao Productions/Stocksy **124-125** Phongpol Saengow/EyeEm/Getty **126-127** Dougal Waters/Getty **128-129** Momentimages/Getty **130-131** PeopleImages/Getty **132-133** From left: Tetra Images/Getty; Westend61/Getty **134-135** Brooke Lark/@brookelark/Unsplash **136-137** Skynesher/Getty **138-139** Mediaphotos/Getty **140-141** Miguel De Jesus Gaytan Juarez/EyeEm/Getty **142-143** From left: Courtesy Laurie Lewis; Surachet99/Getty **144-145** From left: Melissa Ross/Getty; RicoWde/Getty **146-147** Tenkende/Getty **148-149** Jayme Thornton/Getty **150-151** From left: Fascinadora/Getty; Deagreez/Getty **152-153** Orbon Alija/Getty **154-155** Ersinkisacik/Getty **156-157** Towfiqu Photography/Getty **158-159** Seksak Kerdkanno/EyeEm/Getty **160-161** Marc Tran/Getty **162-163** Pascal Broze/Getty **164-165** From left: Btkstudio/Getty; Portishead1/Getty **166-167** From left: Ken Goodman Photography (2) **168-169** Clockwise from bottom left: Michael Stewart/Getty; Enrique Diaz/7cero/Getty; Jacqueline Byers; Anna Pelzer/@annapelzer/Unsplash **170-171** From left: Nicolas Bets/Getty; Courtesy Rachel Sharp **172-173** Clockwise from left: Madlyinlovewithlife/Getty; Courtesy Andy Aupperle; Topotishka/Shutterstock **174-175** Clockwise from top left: Kedsanee/Getty; Michelle Lee Photography/Shutterstock; Courtesy Ali Bruch **176-177** From left: Christian Vierig/Getty; Roy Rochlin/Getty **178-179** From left: Frazer Harrison/Getty; C Flanigan/Getty; Dimitrios Kambouris/Getty; Axelle/Bauer-Griffin/Filmmagic/Getty (2) **180-181** From left: Simone Comi/Venezia/IPA/Shutterstock; Matt Baron/Shutterstock; George Pimentel/Wireimage/Getty; AFF-USA/Shutterstock **182-183** Kristin Lee/Getty **184-185** Kristin Lee/Getty **INSIDE BACK COVER** Yulkapopkova/Getty **BACK COVER** Clockwise from top left: Sergey Skleznev/Getty; LdF/Getty; LauriPatterson/Getty; Aleksandra Voinova/Shutterstock; Courtesy Rachel Sharp

---

**SPECIAL THANKS TO CONTRIBUTING WRITER KIMBERLY GOAD**

---

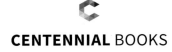

# **CENTENNIAL** BOOKS

An Imprint of
Centennial Media, LLC
40 Worth St., 10th Floor
New York, NY 10013, U.S.A.

ISBN 978-1-951274-50-4

Distributed by
Simon & Schuster, Inc.
1230 Avenue of the Americas
New York, NY 10020, U.S.A.

For information about custom editions, special sales and premium and corporate purchases,
please contact Centennial Media at contact@centennialmedia.com.

Manufactured in China

**Publishers & Co-Founders** Ben Harris, Sebastian Raatz
**Editorial Director** Annabel Vered
**Creative Director** Jessica Power
**Executive Editor** Janet Giovanelli
**Deputy Editors** Ron Kelly, Alyssa Shaffer
**Design Director** Martin Elfers
**Senior Art Director** Pino Impastato
**Art Directors** Runyon Hall, Natali Suasnavas, Joseph Ulatowski
**Copy/Production** Patty Carroll, Angela Taormina
**Assistant Art Director** Jaclyn Loney
**Photo Editor** Keri Pruett
**Production Manager** Paul Rodina
**Production Assistant** Alyssa Swiderski
**Editorial Assistant** Tiana Schippa
**Sales & Marketing** Jeremy Nurnberg